BIRTH WITHOUT VIOLENCE

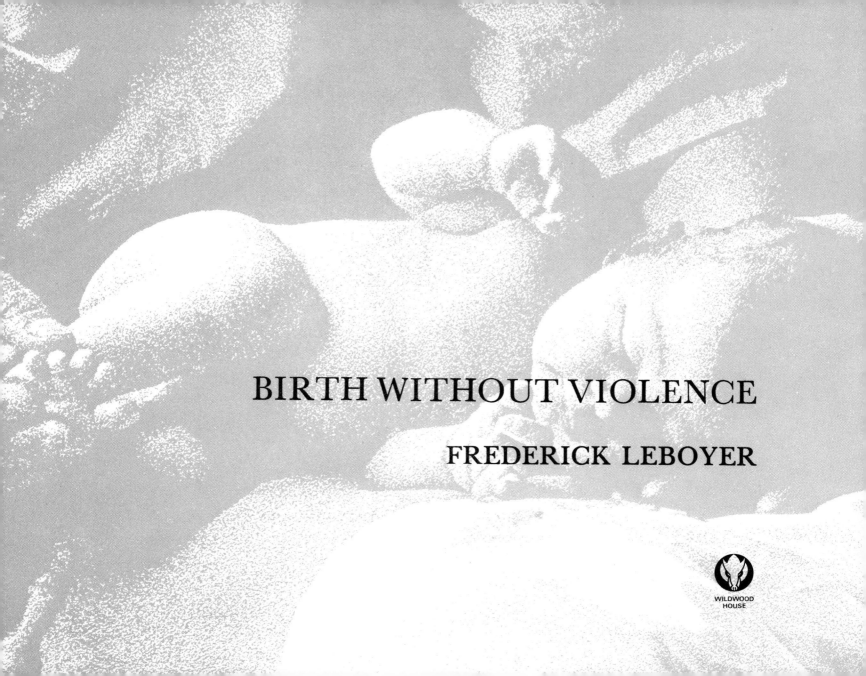

BIRTH WITHOUT VIOLENCE

FREDERICK LEBOYER

WILDWOOD
HOUSE

Originally published in France as *Pour Une Naissance Sans Violence* by
Editions du Seuil, Paris
Copyright © 1974 by Editions du Seuil
Translation copyright © 1975 by Wildwood House Limited

This translation first published in Great Britain 1975 by
Wildwood House Limited, 29 King Street, London WC2

Reprinted 1975

ISBN 0 7045 0171 6

Photographs: pages iii, 29, 30, 39, 40, 51, 53, 57, 58, 78–81, 87, 89, 91, 92, 103, 105 by
Pierre-Marie Goulet; pages 1, 2, 6, 8, 9, 49, 56, 61, 67, 69, 70, 72, 73, 75–77, 83, 85, 88, 104 by
Fréderic Leboyer; pages 11, 12, 20 were supplied by I.M.S., Stockholm

Printed in Great Britain by Biddles Ltd, Guildford, Surrey

BIRTH WITHOUT VIOLENCE

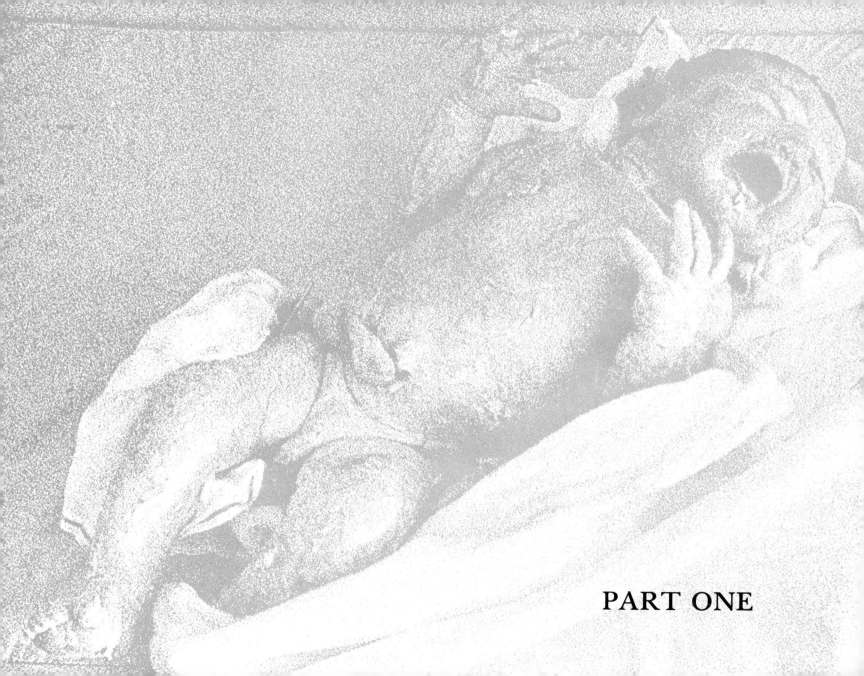

PART ONE

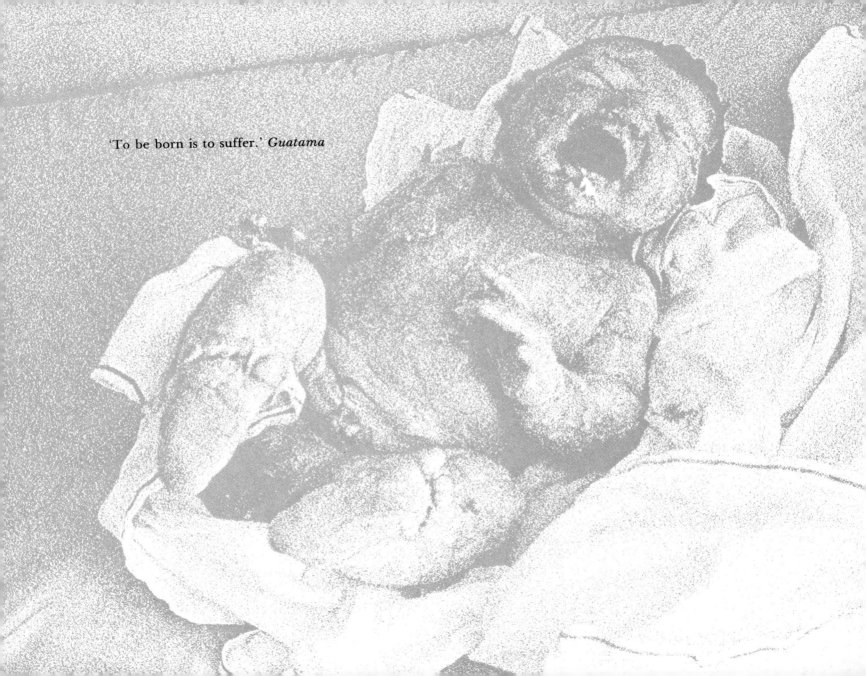

'To be born is to suffer.' *Guatama*

1

'Do you believe that birth is an enjoyable experience . . . for the baby?'

'Birth? Enjoyable?'

'You heard me . . . do you believe that babies feel happy coming into this world?'

'You're joking.'

'Why should I be joking?'

'Because babies are just babies.'

'What is that supposed to mean?'

'That babies aren't capable of intense feelings.'

'What makes you so certain?'

'Babies don't have fully developed feelings.'

'How do you *know*?'

'Well, don't you agree?'

'If I did, I wouldn't be asking.'

'But everybody knows they don't.'

'Since when has that ever been a good reason to believe anything?'

'True. But newborn babies can't see or even hear, so how can they feel unhappy?'

'Even if they can't see or hear, that doesn't stop them from crying their hearts out.'

'A baby has to test its lungs. That's common knowledge.'

'Nonsense!'

'Well, that's what people say.'

'People say all kinds of stupid things. But do you really believe that babies feel nothing at all while they're being born?'

'Obviously they don't.'

'I'm not so sure. After all, young children suffer overwhelming agonies about things that seem quite trivial to us — they feel a thousand times more intensely than we do.'

'Yes, I know, but newborn babies are so tiny.'

'What does size have to do with it?'

'Well . . .'

'And why do they scream so loud if they're not in some kind of pain or misery?'

'I don't know — a reflex I suppose. But I'm sure they're not feeling anything.'

'But *why* aren't they?'

'Because they have no conscious awareness.'

'Ah. So you think that means they have no soul.'

'I don't know about the soul.'

'But this consciousness . . . why is it so important?'

'Consciousness is the beginning of being a person.'

'Are you trying to tell me that babies aren't fully human because they're not fully conscious? Tell me more . . . '

2

How many times have I heard that kind of discussion. It leads nowhere. Things are simple. It's we who complicate them.

When children come into the world, the first thing they do is cry. And everyone relaxes.

'Just listen to that,' the mother exclaims happily, astonished that something so small can make so much noise. Traditionally, this crying means that the reflexes are normal, that the machine works.

But are we machines?

Aren't cries always an expression of pain?

Could it not be that the baby is in anguish?

Could it not be that birth is as painful for the child as giving birth once was for the mother?

And if it is, does anyone care?

I'm afraid, judging by how little consideration we give to a baby, apparently not.

We have a sadly deep-rooted prejudice against believing that this 'thing' can feel, hear or see.

So how could it feel pain?

'It' shrieks, it howls, and that is that.

In short, it is an object.

But what if it were already a *person*?

3

Already a person! That would be a contradiction of everything we believe.

Common sense suggests we begin by looking at the facts.

But here they tell us absolutely nothing.

Because babies can't actually 'tell' us anything. They don't speak in words.

Nor do porpoises. Or birds. But that doesn't prevent *them* from communicating.

Are there languages without words? Of course. We know there are, only our vanity keeps us from acknowledging them. Just watch someone accidentally swallow something boiling hot, and you see how eloquently he speaks — and how wordlessly. He leaps up, hops from foot to foot, frantically waving his hands as though to rid himself of the excess heat. His face is contorted, his eyes are watering. Whether he is Eskimo, Turk or Japanese he has managed to say 'I've burned myself' — and to say it without using a single word.

And, compared to being born, burning your mouth is nothing. If there is one thing a newborn baby doesn't lack, it's the ability to express itself.

Let us take a closer look.

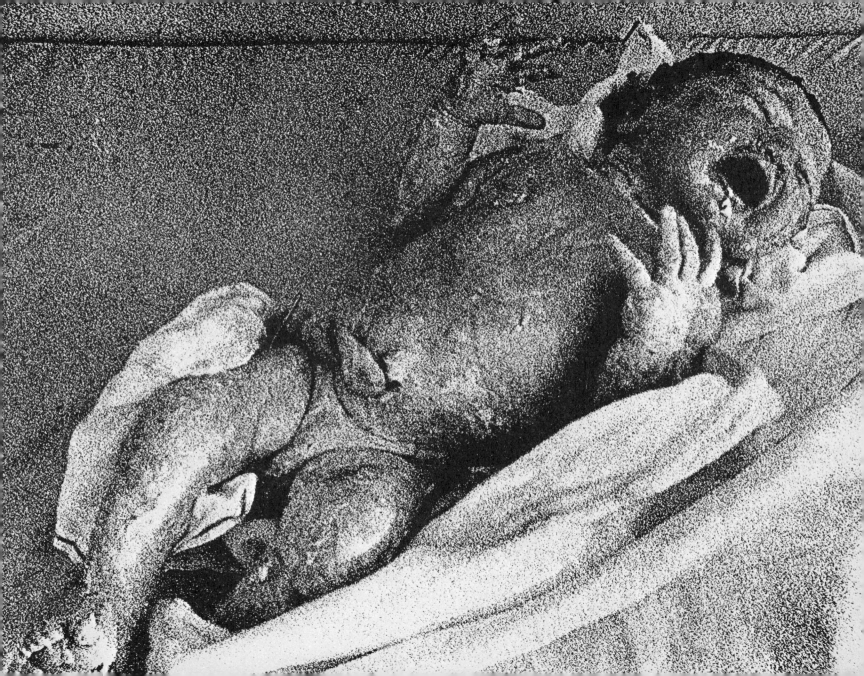

4

The evidence is there before us.

The tragic expression, those tight-shut eyes, those puzzled eyebrows...

That howling mouth, that burrowing, desperate head.

Those outstretched hands beseeching; then withdrawn, raised to the head in the classic gesture of despair.

Those furiously kicking feet, those knees drawn up to protect the tender bulging stomach.

The whole creature is one jumping, twitching mass.

Far from not speaking, every inch of its body is crying out: 'Don't touch me!'

And at the same time pleading: 'Don't leave me! Help me!'

Has there ever been a more heart-rending appeal?

And yet this appeal — as old as birth itself — has been misunderstood, ignored, indeed unheard.

How can this have been? How can this still be?

So can we say that a newborn baby doesn't speak?

No. It is we who do not listen.

5

And so we begin to wonder.

Could this little creature already be a person?

Suffering? Howling with grief?

But it's so young . . . so small . . .

Again something in us resists, doesn't want to hear, refuses to believe.

Something tells us to close our eyes, to safeguard our precious peace of mind.

Clearly we find it intolerable to look . . . to see . . .

Pictures of newly born babies are horrible; they look like tortured prisoners.

People turn away and say: "No! I can't stand it.'

Or: 'Suffering? Do you really think so?'

What you won't see can't hurt you.

Others comment pedantically: 'Birth isn't like that, or we'd know about it. You're showing us a baby being tortured. A baby in the hands of sadists.'

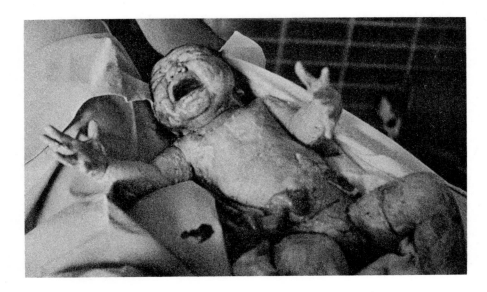

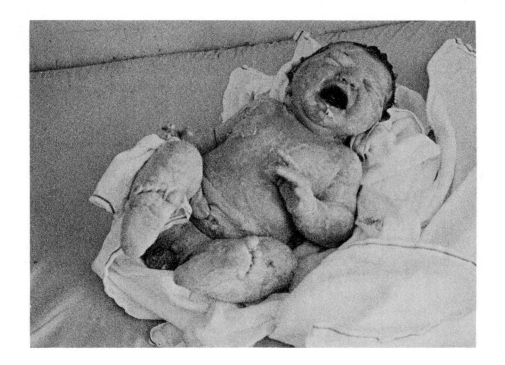

No. Not at all.

It's just a birth.

No monsters, no sadists. Just people like you and me. People whose minds are elsewhere.

'They have eyes but do not see.'

Blind men and women whose eyes are open wide. And we can watch them at it.

6

A small creature has just been born. The father and mother gaze at it with rapture. Even the young assistant looks pleased.

One dazzling smile lights up their faces. They radiate happiness.

All of them, that is, except the child.

The child?

Oh, dear God, it can't be true!

The mask of agony, of horror; and above all the hands, raised to the head . . .

This is the gesture of someone dumbfounded. The gesture of the mortally wounded, the moment before they collapse.

Can birth hold so much suffering, so much pain? While the parents look on in ecstasy, oblivious.

It seems unbelievable.

And yet it's so.

7

Why is the doctor smiling, why does he look so pleased?

For the child? Not really.

He's completed 'his' delivery. He's succeeded at something that's not always easy. The baby is there, crying loudly, as it's supposed to. The mother is safe. Everything has gone well.

The doctor smiles with relief. He is justifiably pleased . . . with himself!

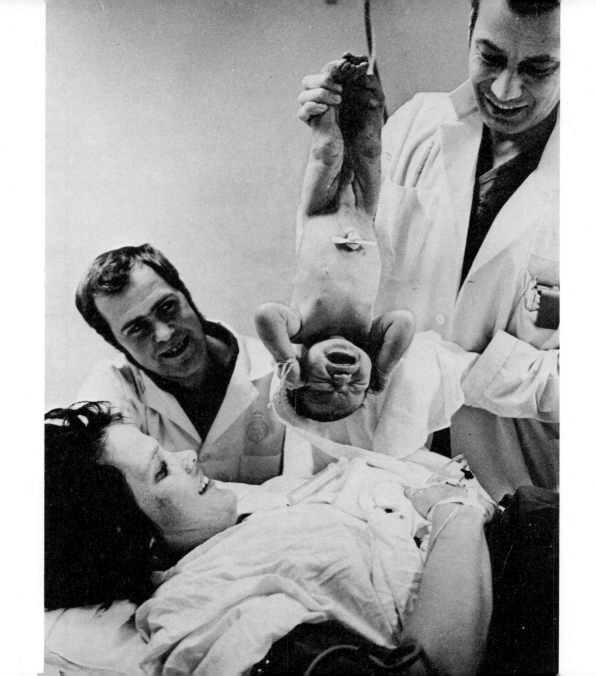

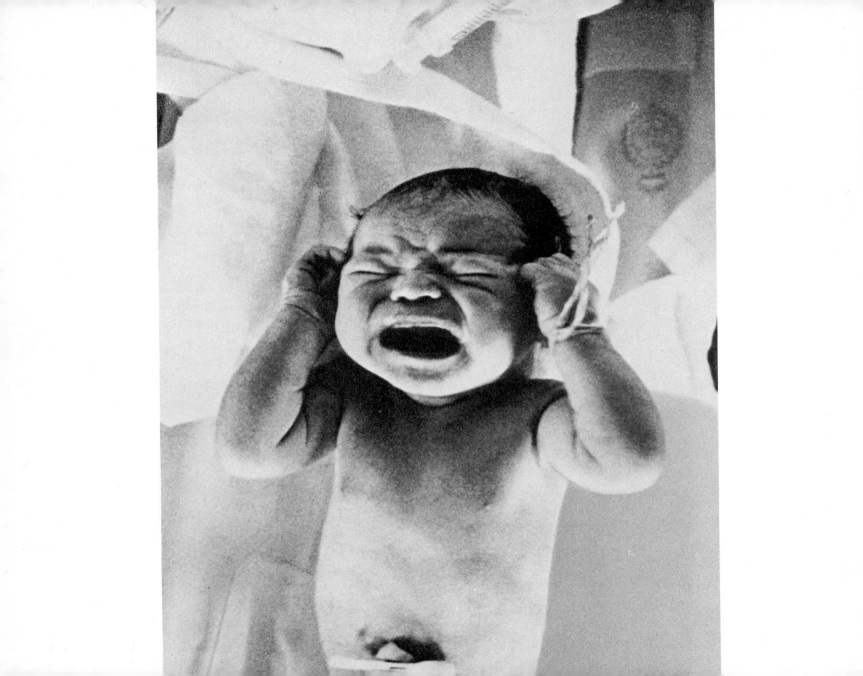

What about the mother?

Radiant expression, ecstatic smile. But what is she smiling about? The beauty of her child? Not really.

She's smiling because it's over.

She has completed 'her' natural childbirth; she had been only half-convinced by the phrase, so she's amazed. And relieved. And — justifiably — proud of herself.

She's smiling with delight.

She's pleased . . . with *herself*.

And who can blame her?

Finally, what about the father?

A happy man. His perfect qualities are now assured of longer life: the baby will grow up to be a replica of its faultless father.

This man, who may never before have truly created anything, has created a child.

And so he is proud. And pleased. But pleased with *himself*. Yes, everyone is pleased. With themselves.

As for the child . . .

8

Should we wring our hands at such suffering, or rather at such blindness?

'You shall give birth in pain,' says the Bible.

But today a woman can give birth joyfully.

Yet how can she be so radiant while her child is still racked with such suffering? It should not be possible.

Should the woman then renounce her joy?

No, certainly not.

We must simply now do for the child what we have already done for the mother. Or at least we must try.

9

Where can we begin?

The mother has to be taught about natural childbirth. But how can we prepare the child? And when? While it is still in the womb?

Are fine electrodes an answer, inserted into the tiny skull through the mother's stomach?

For God's sake, no. Although, these days, technology could achieve such things.

But that is not *our* way.

We must begin by understanding.

Understand *why* the newborn baby suffers so much.

The answer is contained in the question. And to ask: 'Why do babies suffer while being born?' is to open our ears at last to what they have been crying out so desperately for so long.

We must listen to them, we must try to hear, to understand. And we shall be halfway there.

10

What makes being born so frightful is the intensity, the vastness and variety of the experience; its stifling richness.

People say — and believe — that a newborn baby feels nothing. He feels *everything*.

Everything — utterly, without choice or filter or discrimination.

Birth is a tidal wave of sensation, surpassing anything we can imagine.

A sensory experience so huge we can barely conceive of it.

The baby's senses are at work. Totally.

They have the sharpness and freshness of absolute youth.

What are our senses compared to theirs?

And the sensations of birth are made still more intense by contrast with what life was like before; because the senses were already at work long before the baby was here, among us, in our world.

Admittedly, these sensations are not yet organized into integrated, coherent perceptions. But this makes them all the stronger, all the more violent, unbearable, bewildering.

11

Let us begin with sight.

It is claimed that a newborn baby is blind.

Judging by the abundance of blinding lights that are used during deliveries everywhere, this must be a universal postulate.

Glaring lights are mercilessly trained upon the new arrival.

Of course. Who would dim lights for a blind man?

These lights are certainly convenient for the obstetrician.

But what about the baby?

When the baby's head is barely out of its mother's genital passage, while its body is still captive, you see the eyes opening. And shutting again. Immediately and firmly. A look of utter anguish appears on the face and the familiar cry bursts out.

If 'seeing' means making mental images out of what the eyes are exposed to, then indeed the newborn baby doesn't see. At least, probably not.

But if seeing is perceiving light, the baby does see.

Vividly.

The baby has the same love, the same thirst for light that plants and flowers have.

The baby is passionate about light, drunk with it. So much so that we should offer it infinitely slowly, with endless precautions.

In fact, babies are so sensitive to light that they perceive it while still in the mother's womb.

If a woman more than six months' pregnant is naked in the sunlight, the baby within her sees it as a golden haze.

And now this small creature, so sensitive to light, is suddenly thrust out of its dark lair, and its eyes are exposed to floodlights.

It screams, and not surprisingly: its eyes will be smarting almost like those of the people in Hiroshima when 'a thousand suns' broke out.

If our aim were actually to drive it mad with pain, we couldn't go about it better.

The poor baby squeezes its eyes shut. But what help is the fragile, transparent barrier of its eyelids?

The truth is that the newborn baby is not blind, but blinded.

12

And what about hearing? Is the poor baby deaf?

It is no more deaf than blind.

By the time babies are actually born, their ears have already been serving them for some time.

While they were still in the womb, they could hear the noises of their mothers' bodies: joints cracking, tummy rumblings, all backed by the strong drumbeat of the mother's heart.

Not to mention her voice. The mother's voice, which sets its stamp upon the children for ever.

Each voice is as unique and inimitable as a set of fingerprints.

The unborn baby is marked by its mother's voice, its nuances, its inflections, its moods.

Furthermore, just as they perceive light, unborn babies perceive the sounds of the world — despite the thickness of the mother's stomach wall.

They receive them, modulated, transformed, the way fish do, through the waters in which they bathe.

At birth, sounds — muted until now — suddenly strike with all their force. The waters have vanished; the protective shield of the mother's stomach is gone.

Now the baby's ears are suddenly vulnerable, unprotected from the world's uproar.

The baby is born into a thunderous explosion. It is thoroughly alarmed. Should we be surprised?

The world seems to be roaring. The child roars back.

Once again, it is we who are deaf. Our ears, assailed by the sounds of a lifetime, no longer hear anything at all.

No one bothers to lower their voice in the delivery room. In fact, people shout there rather than speak.

'Come on! Keep pushing! Again, again!'

And in the general excitement, when the child emerges, what it hears is exclamations, new explosions of sound.

How does the child react?

Again, by cradling its head in its hands, as though in crippling pain.

So, is the newborn baby deaf?

No. Stunned.

13

Poor creature! What a fate, to be born and to fall straight into the lap of our ignorance and cruelty.

It has been blinded and deafened.

What about its sense of touch?

Its skin — thin, fine, almost without a protective surface layer — is as exposed and raw as tissue that has suffered a burn. The slightest touch makes it quiver.

A newborn baby even trembles when someone comes near it. Until birth, its skin knew only the uniform smoothness of membrane. Then, suddenly, it is put in nappies, shawls, sheets.

Newborn babies arrive in our world as if on a briar patch.

They will adapt to it.

And here, as elsewhere, adaptation means withdrawal, deadening of the senses.

But when they first land on these thorns, they howl.

Naturally.

And, idiots that we are, we laugh.

But this is just the beginning.

14

Hell exists, and is white-hot. It is not a fable.

But we go through it at the beginning of our lives, not at the end.

Hell is what the child goes through to reach us.

Its flames assail the child from every side; they burn its eyes, its skin, they sear its flesh; they devour.

This fire is what the baby feels as the air rushes into the lungs.

The air, which enters and sweeps through the trachea, and expands the alveoli, is like acid poured on a wound.

This is no exaggeration. We have only to watch someone trying to inhale cigarette smoke for the first time. It's nothing to the habitual smoker — his saturated membranes have long ago given up the battle. But the novice, whose tissues are still reasonably undamaged, no sooner takes a lungful of smoke than he explodes in a frantic effort to be rid of its intolerable burning. His eyes water, his face turns crimson.

Or imagine a child who, fooled by the colourlessness of pure alcohol, accidentally drinks it in place of water.

No sooner does it reach the child's throat than it is vomited back up in a single violent reaction, while tears mingle with shuddering and hiccups, and he turns scarlet.

For the baby coming into this world, the burning sensation of air entering the lungs is the worst horror of all.

Seared to its very depths, the entire body quivers, shudders with horror, protests.

Everything struggles to drive the enemy out.

And this is the baby's cry!

The cry that marks and celebrates the passage into life. It is a 'No.' A passionate, violent protest. A cry that is as desperate as it is useless.

For this is only the first of all the many breaths that are to follow — and each burns more than the one before.

15

And is *this* all?

Alas, no.

When the baby emerges, the doctor seizes it by one foot and holds it dangling, head down.

As usual, his intentions are good.

The baby's body is, in fact, very slippery, coated as it is with *vernix caseosa,* the thick, white grease that covers it from head to toe. The baby is held by the foot to prevent it from slipping and falling. Such a hand-hold is sure. Convenient.

Convenient for *us*.

And for the baby?

How does it feel, finding itself suddenly hanging like that?

Indescribably dizzy.

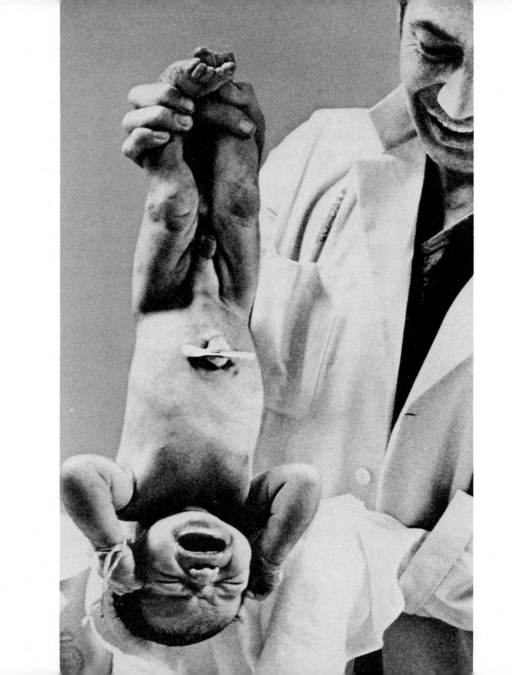

Those who have had nightmares in which they suddenly plunge into nothingness are familiar with this sensation. It stems directly from this moment during their birth.

To understand the full horror of such a fall into the abyss, it is essential that we go back for a moment to the mother's womb.

So little attention do we pay our bodies, that we forget the importance of our own back.

It is 'behind' us. Yet it rules our every mood — whether energetic and cheerful or limp and gloomy.

We say 'put your back into it' and talk of people 'shouldering' responsibilities. Our states of mind are really states of back! And to understand the horror of the shock we inflict on a baby when we suspend it over nothingness, we must first grasp what the back is undergoing at that moment. We must measure the difference between its 'before' and its 'now'. 'Before' was what the backbone experienced when, with great difficulty, the baby was trying to find its way out into the world.

In fact, we must go back even further, into the mother's uterus. And there we must re-live what this back has undergone.

16

A baby's life passes through two stages in the womb: two seasons of equal length, but as different as winter from summer.

The first is 'the golden age'.

The embryonic stage, when the infant is like a small plant, growing and blossoming.

Anchored.

The embryo becomes the foetus; the plant becomes animal.

It breaks out into gentle movement, beginning at the trunk, spreading outwards to the extremities.

The foetus takes pleasure in its limbs. And in its freedom.

Buoyed up by waters around it, the foetus is weightless, light as a bird, agile and lively as a fish.

Its contentment and freedom are limitless. And its kingdom, whose boundaries it brushes from time to time, is vast indeed.

For in this first half of pregnancy, the egg (the membrane which contains the foetus and the fluids in which it is bathed) grows more rapidly than the child.

Fast as the child develops, its kingdom grows faster.

So the baby never suffers a sense of confinement.

The photographs we have of it at this stage show a completely relaxed expression.

A vision of serenity.

This is the Golden Age.

But it doesn't last.

In the depths of the womb, the child has been overtaken by Natural Law. The law of universal revolution, which decrees that everything, ultimately, must become its opposite.

Midway through pregnancy, everything changes. The child continues to grow and to develop rapidly. But the egg that contains it grows only slightly by comparison.

Its tribulations begin.

The baby begins to feel closed in; slowly, insidiously, its universe is contracting.

What was once unbounded space becomes more confining each day. Gone is the limitless ocean of earlier — and happier — days; that absolute freedom is no more.

And one day the baby finds itself . . . a prisoner.

And what a prison!

The cell so small that the prisoner's body touches all the walls at once. The walls close in upon it all the time. Until, one day, the child's back and the mother's uterus seem to be fused together.

For a long time, the child won't accept it. It struggles and protests.

In vain. Inexorably the prison closes in.

It bows its head and curls up into a ball.

Perhaps some instinct suggests to it that nothing lasts for ever, that perhaps its present suffering may be rewarded by future joys. It resigns itself; indeed, it has no choice.

Each day the baby grows larger inside the shrinking prison.

It huddles up. It crouches and submits.

Then one day the prison comes to life. No longer content merely to keep the child huddled in submission, it begins, like some octopus, to hug and crush.

Terrified, the child endures.

The contraction ceases, returns, ebbs . . . then there is another.

Not strong, more like a game.

So that once the child has recovered from its initial fright, it becomes accustomed to the contractions, and even begins to like them.

They are, after all, a diversion.

When they come — hugging the child firmly — it surrenders to them; arches its back, quivers with pleasure at this sensual game.

This dalliance lasts throughout the whole of the ninth month. Painless for the mother, it prepares the child for the contractions of actual labour, which will be ten times more intense.

17

One day, these contractions are no longer a game. They crush, they stifle, they assault.

One day labour starts. The delivery has begun.

Now the child is in the grip of a huge, frenzied, intransigent force.

Curling up is no longer the answer.

Helpless, it huddles up even more tightly. With its head tucked in and its shoulders hunched, it is a compact ball of fright.

The prison has gone beserk, and seems bent on its inmate's

destruction. The walls close in still further. The cell narrows hatefully, and becomes a funnel.

Its heart bursting, the child is thrust into this hell.

Then, suddenly, fear changes to anger.

Enraged, the child hurls itself against the barrier.

At all costs, it must break through. Free itself.

Yet all this force, this monstrous unremitting pressure that is crushing the baby, pushing it out towards the world, and this blind, blank wall, which is holding it back, confining it — these things are all one: the mother!

She is driving her baby out.

At the same time she is holding it in, blocking its passage.

It is *she* who is the enemy. She who stands between the child and life.

Only one of them can prevail, it is a fight to the death.

The child is like a soul possessed.

Mad with agony and misery, alone, abandoned, it fights on with the strength of despair.

The monster drives the baby lower still. Not satisfied with crushing it, she twists it in a refinement of cruelty.

To negotiate the narrow passage of the pelvis, the baby's head and body execute a corkscrew-like motion as though in a wine-press.

It seems incredible that the child's head — bearing the brunt of the struggle until it is almost forced down between the shoulder blades, down on to the chest — should withstand it at all.

The baby is now at the height of its travail. The effort required is too great. The end is surely near. Death seems certain.

The monster bears down one more time . . .

18

It is then that everything explodes!

The whole world bursts open.
No more tunnel, no prison, no monster.
The child is born.
Where are those walls? Vanished, pushed away.
Nothing!
Instead, there is emptiness and all its horrors.
Freedom! — and it is intolerable.
Where am I . . .
I was cramped and stifled, but at least I had a form.
My mother, my hated prison — where are you?
Alone, I am nothingness, dizziness.
Take me back! Enclose me. Crush me, destroy me.
But let me exist . . .

19

The child feels an obscure anguish: for the first time, its back is unsupported.

And it is in this paroxysm of confusion, of despair and distress, that someone seizes the baby by a foot and lets it hang over the void.

The spinal column has been strained, bent, pushed and twisted to the limit of its endurance — and now it is left to its own devices.

And the head, so supremely involved in the passage outwards, is now felt feebly dangling in thin air.

And this is happening at the very moment when in order to soothe this vast terror, this panic, what is essential is that the whole body should be collected, pressed, held together.

If our deliberate intention were to teach the child that it had fallen into an indifferent world, a world of ignorance, cruelty and folly, what better course of action could we have chosen?

20

Now, where do we place the terrified baby, who has so painfully emerged from the enveloping warmth and softness of the womb?

On the scales.

Sometimes even steel scales, cold with a cold that burns like fire.

The crying mounts.

And so does the joy of the onlookers.

Particularly if the baby's weight, when it is announced, is impressive.

'It certainly knows how to cry!' the ecstatic mother says.

The baby is picked up again.

Again by the feet, head dangling.

More dizziness and terror.

The baby is laid down again. On any nearby surface, among the bits and pieces that accompany babyhood.

It is abandoned, still crying.

Then there are its eyes to see to, drops to be given.

The baby struggles.

Its eyes are forced open.

And several tears of burning liquid are dropped in.

21

And now the baby is alone.

Abandoned by everyone and everything, lost in a world as hostile as it is incomprehensible. Still trembling with terror. Hiccuping, choking.

Unhappiness is so ingrained in most babies by this time that they hope for nothing else.

They tremble like leaves at the mere approach of a human being.

And then we see an extraordinary thing: when the tears and gasping and the distress become too much, the baby escapes.

Not literally of course; its legs will not help it.

The baby disappears into itself.

It doubles up again, and curls up into a ball, folding its arms and legs around itself.

It has once again adopted the foetal position, the posture of past unhappiness.

Symbolically, it has taken itself back into the womb.

Overcome by the horror of the world, it returns to paradise. It objects to having been born. It becomes a foetus again. And once again . . . a prisoner.

22

Calm.

But not for long.

The baby is picked up again and dressed.

In things that are tight, rough, heavy; but which 'look so pretty'. Which please the mother, family and friends . . . Once again the baby protests, bursts into loud sobs, cries, shrieks.

For as long as its considerable strength holds out.

And when it is no longer able to cry, it collapses.

It subsides into sleep.

Its only refuge.

Its only friend.

23

Such is birth.

The torture of an innocent.

One would have to be naive indeed to believe that so great a cataclysm would not leave its mark.

Its traces are everywhere; on the skin, in the bones, in the stomach, in the back, in all our human folly, in our madness, our tortures, our prisons, in legends, epics and in myths. The scriptures themselves are surely none other than this abominable tale of woe.

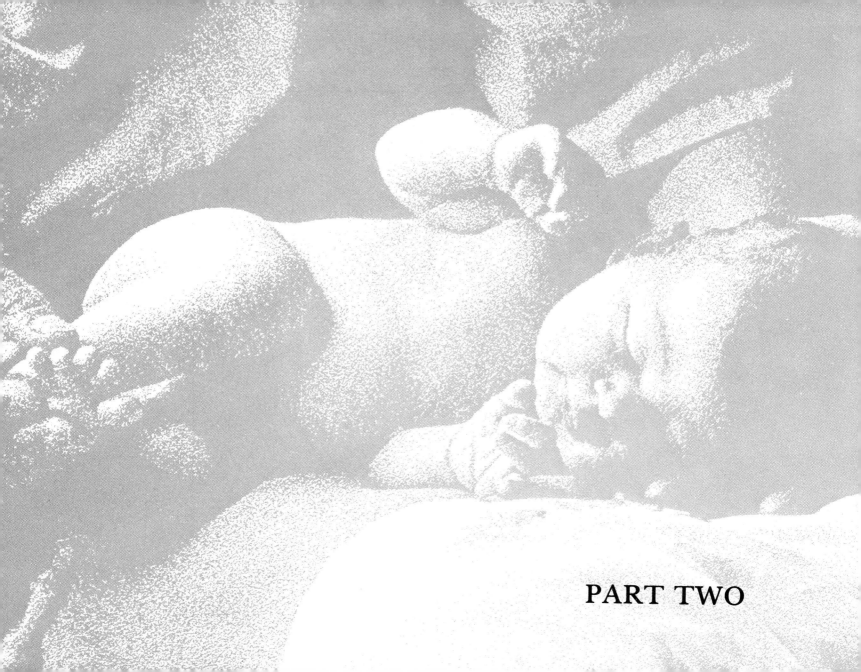

PART TWO

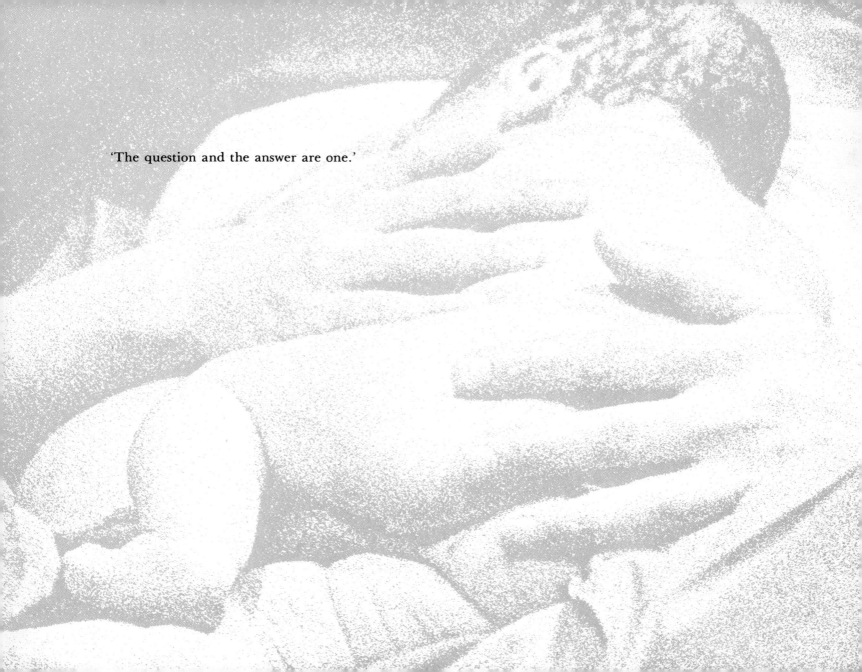

'The question and the answer are one.'

1

All of this is terrifying, overwhelming; it leaves us almost without hope.

Without hope for the child.

Should we prepare the child while still in the womb? With electrodes?

No, it isn't the child who needs preparation. It is we ourselves.

If we manifest such blindness, so little understanding in the way we welcome newborn children, can we marvel that the world is . . . the way it is?

For the moment, let us concentrate on the process of birth.

Let us see how even a modest increase of sensitivity on our part can make an immense difference.

2

There is a disquieting paradox in birth.

The child suddenly finds itself liberated from an unendurable captivity . . . and shrieks!

This also happens, apparently, to prisoners who are suddenly set free.

The freedom they have dreamt of so long intoxicates them — and makes them panic.

They begin to miss their prison bars. Both better off and worse off than before, unconsciously they behave in ways that will ensure them re-imprisonment.

In the same way, the baby howls, choked with freedom.

Irritated, we want to say: 'But this is absurd, you ought to be babbling with delight, not crying. Now at last you can unwind, stretch, kick, wave your arms; and yet you're crying! Look around you. Observe your kingdom and your happiness.'

It must be made to understand; it must listen to reason.

Reason? A tiny creature only a few minutes old? Few enough people listen to reason at the best of times. Then *how* can we tell the baby?

'Tell' is not the right word.

We must talk to the baby in its own language, the language that precedes words.

Are we then, to speak in gestures, as we would to a foreigner?

Of course not.

We must go back still further and rediscover the universal language, which is simply the language of love.

Can this be right for a newborn baby?

Yes; we must speak of love. We must speak the language of lovers.

And what is the essential language of lovers?

Not speech. Touch.

Lovers are shy, modest, When they want to make contact in their particular way, they seek the darkness; they turn out the light. Or simply close their eyes.

They create night around them. The other senses are blacked out. Touch becomes everything.

And in this newfound darkness, they put their arms around each other, to recreate that old, beloved prison, they are silent; they do not need words.

At most, they might sigh with pleasure.

It is their hands that speak.

And their bodies listen and understand.

This is what newborn babies need. This is how we should speak to them, this is how they understand; simply by tenderness, by touch.

Taking the senses one by one, let us see what we can do so as not to terrify the child who has come among us.

3

It is really quite simple.

Let us begin with the problem of sight.

And put ourselves, like lovers, in the dark.

Now our alertness, our sense of touch, grow keener. But, above all, the child's eyes will be spared.

Of course some light is necessary to attend to the mother, so that she will not be injured when the child's head emerges. But strong lights are unnecessary.

As soon as the head appears and the danger has passed, we should turn out all the lights, except a small night light. That is quite enough.

In the half-darkness, the mother will only be able to make out her child's features faintly. And this is all to the good, since the features of newborn babies are almost always distorted by fear.

It is better for the mother to discover her child by touching it. Better to feel before she sees. Better to sense this warm trembling life; to be thoroughly moved by what her *hands* tell her. To hold her child rather than look at it.

Later she will have plenty of time for that, when its face has relaxed into its true features.

This is the moment for her to speak to her baby quietly, to calm it with her touch.

Both of them, mother and child, have everything to gain by first meeting in the semi-darkness.

But mainly it is for the benefit of the child, whose eyes are spared the burning light.

4

Now hearing . . .

Simplicity itself: be silent.

In actual fact, this is not so easy.

Most people are natural chatterers; and even when we're not actually talking we ramble on inwardly.

Besides, to be silent in someone else's company is so disturbing that we rarely like to attempt it.

To be silent, attentive, to *listen*, to hear that which is unspoken — all this demands great effort, indeed it needs positive training.

The first women whose babies were delivered in silence were so disconcerted by it that their story is worth telling. We were talking very little, and quietly, during the last stages of labour and during the birth itself. The idea was to create a peaceful atmosphere.

And when the children were born, we did not speak a single word.

If occasionally it was absolutely necessary to say something — to give orders or instructions — it was done in an all but inaudible whisper, so as not to disturb each child's first moments.

This procedure — completely natural and yet so unusual — so disturbed the mothers that they quickly became panic-stricken.

Instead of howling as expected, each baby merely uttered two or three healthy cries and then contented itself with powerful breathing. So that in the intense silence that followed, what each woman heard was the very absence of her baby's cry. Her eyes soon betrayed first surprise and then alarm, darting questioningly from one of us to the next.

At last, unable to restrain themselves, each burst out: 'Why isn't my baby crying?' They seemed positively aggrieved. The surprise, the regret, the *accusation* in those questions dumbfounded us. We had not realized

34

how deeply ingrained is the assumption that the newborn child must cry, how profound the unconscious acceptance that birth and suffering are one.

What could we say? What should we tell them?

These women had not been sufficiently forewarned or prepared for this silence, so rare and yet so natural.

We have come so far from the natural life that something as true and simple as this peacefulness can surprise and distress us.

'My baby's dead,' each agonized voice continued.

'Your child is fine,' we said, gesturing to them to lower their voice in order to spare the baby's ears.

Our whispering would upset them still more.

'Dead! My baby's dead!' they said, intoning the old litany.

Dead? Their children were lying on their stomachs, flickering with newborn, undersea movement.

'Now really dead children don't move. Feel your baby moving. Feel how happy he is!' But we were still speaking in the low tones that go with grief.

How can we please both the mother and the child?

And then we tried, admittedly too late, to explain the reason for our silence.

Our respect for the newborn child and its delicate hearing, our determination not to frighten it with sudden noise. We tried to explain to these mothers that crying and suffering are not essential to birth. But our explanations came too late and failed to convince; their eyes were still full of doubt and sorrow.

Finally they grew calmer.

'Your baby is really doing splendidly, as well as a baby can,' we said encouragingly.

'Do you really mean it?' they asked incredulously.

To be fair, we must admit that a newborn baby who begins gurgling happily after just a cry or two — who yawns and stretches, who enters life the way we awake from a restful sleep — is something of a surprise. It is as unexpected, as startling to the uninitiated as is a mother who gives birth smiling, silent and radiant.

So it seems that nowadays we need explanations for what is natural. We must be awake and aware.

Aware that the baby can hear, aware of how sensitive its hearing is, and how easily harmed.

In fact, we must all learn in this first moment to love the baby for itself. Not for ourselves. It is not an extra special possession, to show off.

It is a life entrusted to us, all.

Mothers must begin to feel: 'I am its mother,' and not: 'This is *my child.*'

A world of difference lies between the two.

And the whole future of the child.

5

This apprenticeship of silence — so indispensible for mothers — is just as important for those who perform the delivery: the obstetricians or midwives.

People speak loudly in the delivery room. Encouragements to 'push, push' are rarely whispered, which is a pity.

These roaring exhortations upset the mother rather than help her. Lowered voices can relax her, and do far more for her than shouting.

People involved in deliveries must learn this new silence. They too must be prepared to receive the child with care and respect.

6

With half-darkness and silence, we have created a deeply peaceful world, almost without realizing it.

People don't shout in church. On the contrary, instinctively, they speak quietly. And any room into which a newborn baby comes is at least as worthy of respect.

Darkness and quiet: what else do we need?

Patience. Or more precisely, the learning of an extreme slowness that borders on immobility.

Without this slowness, success is impossible; without it, we cannot communicate with a baby.

Accepting the slow pace, immersing oneself in it — this too requires training. As much for the mother as for those of us who are helping her. Once again, success depends on our understanding the strange world the baby has inhabited so far.

We must remember that his descent into hell proceeded centimetre by centimetre, or more slowly still. As his movements became more and more constricted, they accumulated a considerable store of force and energy.

Without experiencing this extreme slowness in our own bodies, it is impossible to understand birth, and impossible to receive the newborn baby properly.

His rhythm is so slow as to be virtually static.

Ours is an agitation bordering on frenzy.

Besides, we are never truly here — always elsewhere. In the past, with our memories; in the future, with our plans. Always before or after.

Never *now*.

But we must learn to be in the present.

To forget the future and forget the past. → Is HE NO CONCERNED WITH THE FUTURE?

Once again, everything is very simple. And yet so hard to achieve.

How is it to be accomplished?

Only with the most total, unflagging attention.

We who are watching must rediscover the newborn baby, as if this were the first baby we had ever seen. We must be so astounded that we forget everything else. Ourselves included. The age-old division between observer and observed must fade.

We must disappear.

So that only the baby remains.

We must look at this baby. Or better yet, be absorbed into its very being.

Without complications. Without prejudice. In all innocence. All newness.

We must *become* this new person.

But we are looking too far ahead.

Let us wait for the baby.

7

Now.

Everything is ready. Darkness, silence and ourselves.

Time stands still.

The child can make its entrance.

8

Now is the moment.

The baby emerges . . . first the head, and then the arms; we help to free them by sliding a finger under each armpit. Supporting the baby this way, we lift the little body up, as if pulling someone out of a well. We *never* touch the head. And we settle the child immediately on its mother's stomach.

What better place could there be? Her stomach has the baby's exact shape and dimensions. Swelling a moment before, hollow now, the belly

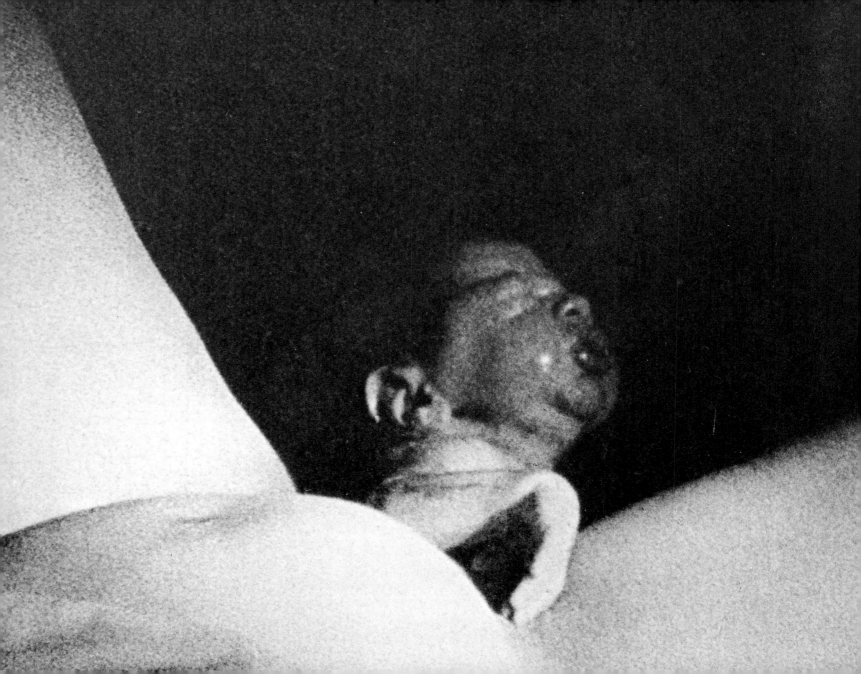

seems to lie there waiting, like a nest.

And its warmth and suppleness as it rises and falls with the rhythm of her breathing, its softness, the warmth of its skin, all make it the best possible resting place for the child.

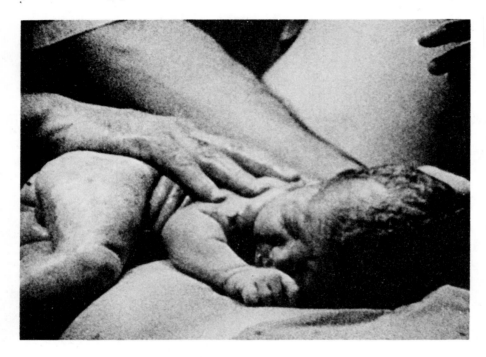

9

To sever the umbilicus when the child has scarcely left the mother's womb is an act of cruelty, whose ill effects are immeasurable. To conserve it intact while it still pulses is to transform the act of birth.

I presume he means the umbilical cord which has no nerve supply.

40

First, this forces the doctor to be patient; it is an invitation to both the doctor and the mother to respect the baby's own life-rhythm.

And it does more.

As we have said, when air rushes into the baby's lungs, it burns like fire.

Before he was born, the baby made no distinction between the world and himself, since 'outside' and 'inside' were all one.

He knew nothing of the tension of opposites — nothing was cold, since cold can only be known by contrast with what is warm. An infant's body temperature and its mother's are naturally always identical; since there is no barrier between the two.

For the newborn child, to enter our world is to enter a realm of opposites, where everything is good or bad, pleasant or unpleasant, dry or wet . . .

These contradictions, it will find, are inextricably intertwined.

And how does the baby enter this realm of opposites? Through breathing. In taking its first breath, it crosses a threshold. And it is here.

The baby takes a breath. And from this inhalation springs its opposite — exhalation.

A pendulum has been released into perpetual motion — the very principle of our world, where everything is breathing, rocking; where everything, always, is born from its opposite — day from night, summer from winter, strength from weakness.

Without end. Without beginning.

10

To breathe is to be in accord with creation, to be in harmony with the Universal, with its eternal pulse. More literally, it is to take in oxygen and to expel the wastes, essentially carbon dioxide.

But in this simple exchange, two worlds approach one another, attempt to touch, to mix, to meet: the world within and the world without.

Two worlds, now separate, try to recover each other, to become one again: the small 'I' inside and the vast world outside.

Both the blood that rises from below, and the air that sweeps in from above, flow into the lungs.

Air and blood rush towards each other, eager to mix.

They are unable to do so, separated as they are by a wall, the thin partition of the alveoli.

And each sighs after their lost unity.

The blood arrives in the lungs — dull, depleted of oxygen, heavy with carbon dioxide and the other waste products that render it old, without vitality, exhausted. In the lungs it will shed its age, and recharge itself with youth and energy.

Transfigured by its visit to this Fountain of Youth, it sets off again, lively, rich and red, it plunges down again to distribute its riches, rises again, burdened with wastes. Returns to the lungs, where it regenerates itself. And the circle continues indefinitely.

As for the heart, it is the prime mover, sending this regenerated blood to the thirsty tissues of the entire organism, along the course of what is called the major or systemic circulatory system. While in an opposed but synchronous movement it draws the old, depleted blood back towards the source of renewal, the lungs. This is known as the minor or pulmonary circulatory system.

The minor circulatory system derives its name from the shortness of the journey the depleted blood makes from the heart to the lungs and back.

The major circulatory system is so called because of the length of the trips the blood makes from the heart to the limits of its realm, the top of the head, the extremities of the limbs, the internal organs.

How do these things take place within the unborn foetus, whose lungs do not yet function?

For its blood, too, must be regenerated.

This is done by the placenta, which functions as its lungs. The blood arrives and leaves the placenta by way of the umbilical cord, which is nothing more than three tubes: a vein and two arteries in a sheath.

The blood regenerates itself in the placenta, not by contact with outside air but by contact with the mother's blood, which is restored in *her* lungs . . . in short: the mother breathes for her baby. Just as she eats for her baby, carries her baby, shelters her baby. Sleeps and dreams and does everything for it.

Before this baby is born, dependence on the mother is total.

And what happens at birth? An extraordinary adventure, an upheaval, a revolution: the blood which until then has flowed through the umbilicus now ventures into the new lungs.

The baby's blood abandons the old, familiar path, the route through the mother.

By breathing — by oxygenating its blood with its own lungs — the baby takes the path of autonomy, of independence, of freedom.

Of course, this is only the first step. For everything but air the child still depends on its mother.

But the first step has been taken.

The blood, however, does not abandon the old route of the umbilicus-placenta promptly and rudely, all at once. It does not hurl itself into the lungs like a mad thing.

Or at least it shouldn't. And this is the crux of the matter.

Depending on whether this transition occurs slowly, gently — or brutally, in panic and terror — birth becomes a peaceful awakening . . . or a tragic one.

11

Nature, it is said, never moves in sudden leaps.

Yet birth is just such a leap. An exchange of worlds, of levels.

How can we resolve this contradiction? How does nature smooth over a transition whose very essence is so violent?

Very simply.

Nature is strict, but loving. We misunderstand her intentions, then blame her for what follows.

Everything about birth is arranged so that both leap and landing can in fact be gentle.

The danger the child faces during birth has quite properly been stressed.

This danger is anoxia: a deficiency of the crucial oxygen to which the nervous system is so acutely sensitive.

If it happens that the child fails to receive oxygen, the result is irreparable damage to the brain: a person maimed for life.

So at all costs, the child must not lack oxygen at birth, not even for an instant.

As the experts tell us.

As nature has always known.

She has arranged it so that during the dangerous process of birth, the child is receiving oxygen from two sources rather than one: from the lungs *and* from the umbilicus.

Two systems function simultaneously, one relieving the other: the old one, the umbilicus, continues to supply oxygen to the baby until the new one, the lungs, has fully taken its place.

However, once the baby has been born and delivered from the mother, it remains bound to her by this umbilicus, which continues to beat for several minutes: four, five, sometimes more.

Oxygenated by the umbilicus, protected from anoxia, the baby can settle into breathing without danger and without shock, unhurried, and in its own time.

In addition, the blood has plenty of time to abandon its old route (which leads to the placenta) and progressively to fill the pulmonary circulatory system.

During this period, moreover, an orifice closes in the heart, which seals off the old route for ever.

44

In short, for an average of four or five minutes, the newborn infant straddles two worlds. Drawing oxygen from two sources, it switches gradually from the one to the other, without a brutal transition, with scarcely a cry.

What is required for this miracle to take place? Only a little patience. Only a refusal to rush things, a willingness to wait; giving the child time to adjust.

Clearly, one needs to know this; otherwise how could we wait five long minutes doing absolutely nothing, when *everything* contributes to our desire to act: our thoughtlessness, our automatic assumptions, our habits, and our perpetual impatience.

12

For the baby, it makes an enormous difference.

Whether we cut the umbilical cord immediately or not changes everything about the way respiration comes to the baby, and so may even condition the baby's feelings about life.

If the cord is severed as soon as the baby is born, the brain is brutally deprived of oxygen.

The alarm system is thus alerted, and the baby's entire organism reacts. Respiration comes into action as a response to aggression.

Everything in the body-language of the child — the frenzied agitation of its limbs, the very tone of its cries — expresses the immensity of its panic and its efforts to escape.

Entering life, what the baby meets is death. And to escape this death it **hurls itself into respiration. For a newborn baby the act of breathing is a** last resort. Already the first conditioned reflex has been implanted, a reflex in which breathing and anguish will be associated for ever. What a start in life.

13

How do things happen when we refrain from interfering and leave the umbilicus?

Doubly supplied with oxygen, the baby's brain is never threatened, even for a minute. Nothing occurs to set off the alarm system. Consequently, no attack, no anoxia, no panic or anguish.

Rather, a slow and gradual progression from one state to another, with the blood changing course without sudden disruption.

The lungs are not convulsed into action.

When the baby emerges, it utters a cry. This is because the thorax — which until now has been thoroughly constricted by external pressure — is suddenly released and opens wide.

A void is created. The air rushes in. This is the first breath, a passive acceptance.

Nonetheless, it burns.

The child responds by breathing out furiously, and this is the cry.

And then, quite often, everything stops.

As if stunned by such pain, the baby pauses.

Sometimes it cries two or three times before pausing.

The pause terrifies us. So we smack, slap, spank.

If we are better trained to control our impulses, trusting in nature and in the steady, continuing pulse of the umbilical cord, we refrain from interfering. And the baby's breathing begins again, by itself. Hesitantly, cautiously at first, still pausing now and again. Still receiving oxygen from the umbilicus, the baby can take its time in discovering just how much of the burning it can tolerate.

A pause, then another breath. The baby is getting used to this sensation and gradually begins to breathe deeply. Soon it is taking pleasure in what a few moments ago was pain.

Soon its breathing is full, regular and peaceful.

The child will have uttered no more than one cry. Or two. Or three. And we will have heard no more than some strenuous gasps — powerful, startled, punctuated by tiny cries — exclamations of surprise and an outburst of energy.

Besides the breathing, we shall hear other noises which the baby makes with its lips, nose and throat.

Lots of noises. A whole language. But no shrieks of terror, no cries of despair, of agony, of hysteria.

When a child comes into the world, it must undoubtedly cry.

But it need not weep.

Enjoying this new experience, the baby easily loses all memory of the world it has just left.

14

Our baby's birth is like an awakening from a good sleep.

Why should a baby cling to the past when it is perfectly content in this new present?

So, when the umbilicus has finally stopped beating we cut it.

Actually, what we cut amounts to nothing. It is a dead link that is ready to fall away of its own accord.

The child has not been torn from its mother; the two have merely separated.

Later — when this child takes its first step, ventures into the world of the vertical — the mother will offer her own firm support.

Still unsteady on its legs, the child will clutch its mother's hand . . . release her, then reach for her, only to let her go again. Until one day, sure of its own legs, it will have no further need of her support, will forget the hand that has been held out for so long.

The hand can then be withdrawn; the child has no more use for it. But what if the mother withdrew her hand while the child was still taking that first step? She might think that in this way she was hastening the child's progress, encouraging its instinct for independence. The odds are that she would be accomplishing the opposite: discouraging, not encouraging the baby.

All of this is equally true of the umbilicus. By not immediately cutting the cord, we let the mother accompany her baby's first steps into the world of breathing. She goes on breathing for them both until the child is safely established in its new domain.

Cutting the umbilicus at the first cry is the same as withdrawing the hand at the first step.

15

We must accord the greatest respect to this fragile moment of birth.

The baby is between two worlds, hesitating on a threshold. It must not be hurried or jostled; it must be allowed to enter at its own pace.

This is an extraordinary moment; it is no longer a foetus, but not yet a newborn baby.

It is no longer inside its mother but she is still breathing for it.

An elusive, ephemeral moment.

This is a moment that must be spent alone.

Because this child is free, and frightened by it.

Don't intrude: stand back. Let time pass.

Grant this moment its slowness, and its gravity.

16

The rest is detail.

Once the respiratory system is functioning, all is well. (Or if it is not, then the damage is irreparable.) THIS IS A DEFEATIST ATTITUDE

But even now the details are of vital importance.

How should one place the child on the mother's stomach?

On its side? Flat on its front? On its back?

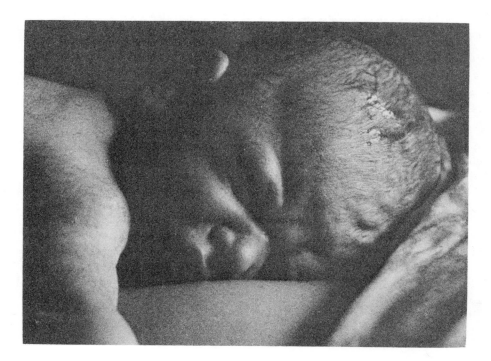

Never on its back. This would cause the spinal column, which has been curved for so long, to straighten at a single go.

The energy that is stored there would be released with such force, such violence, that the shock would be unbearable.

Once again, we must remember that it is necessary to let the child uncurl its spine and stretch its back at its own pace.

Besides, each child is born with its own character, its own temperament.

Some straighten out proudly, arch their backs and stretch their arms (almost as soon as they are born). Their spinal columns straighten out with the force of a tightly strung bow releasing its arrow.

Sometimes, however, shaken by their own temerity, they retract and huddle up again.

Others, tightly curled at first, emerge gradually, venturing out with great caution.

Since we cannot anticipate what is to come, it is best to place the child on its front, arms and legs folded under.

This is the age-old, familiar posture, that best allows the abdomen to breathe freely and permits the baby to work its way (at its own speed) towards the final unbending.

The stretching, the triumphant extension of self.

Moreover, by placing a child on its stomach, we can see its back, watch it in action, observe how it breathes.

In fact, the unbending of the spinal column, the stretching of the back and the start of free respiration are all part of the same process.

Watching this breathing, we can see how it pervades the baby's whole body. Not only its thorax, but its stomach and especially its sides.

Soon the baby appears to be one breathing mass; one sees the powerful waves course up and down its back, from the top of the skull to the coccyx.

And then, cautiously emerging from under the stomach, an arm, usually the right arm.

The arm stretches out. The hand slides briefly over the mother's stomach, then withdraws.

The other hand ventures out . . . slowly, as if astonished to encounter no resistance, surprised that the space around it is so vast . . .

And now the legs begin to move. First one, then the other is cautiously extended. Then both begin to kick and thrash, alarmed because they no longer encounter any resistance.

To calm their panic, we can offer them support; the touch of a hand, offering gentle resistance though letting itself be pushed away.

This overcomes the child's horrible sense of having lost its foothold.

And then, suddenly, everything moves together, harmoniously. There is no part of the little body that is not involved in this movement.

The baby stretches more and more boldly, thrusting, probing. At this

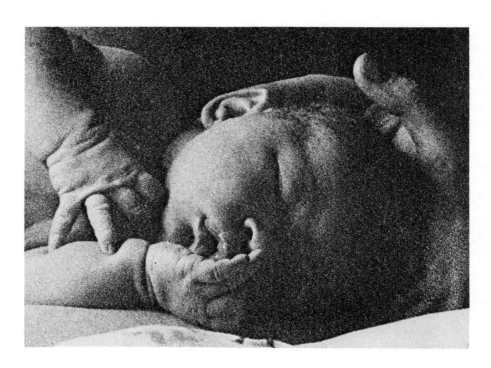

point the child may be placed on its side; its limbs are more relaxed in this position and its spine adopts the posture that is most comfortable for it. We move the baby slowly, always lending support, placing one hand under the baby's bottom, and the other at the top of its back.

It is best not to touch the head, which is extremely sensitive.

This was the part of the child that bore the full weight of the birth drama, of the descent into hell; it was this head that cleared the way. Even the slightest touch can arouse memories that are still too raw.

Finally, when we are sure that everything is functioning well, we put the baby on its back.

. . . Not for long (the baby is still not comfortable with this new straightening of the spine), but simply as a stage of adjustment.

We have taken the edge off the terror. The umbilicus has been cut when it ceased to beat. And we are ready for the next step — to raise this baby upright, into man's privileged vertical posture.

But even now certain precautions are necessary. We must ease the child *slowly* into a sitting position, always supporting the wavering head. The child's own muscles are not yet strong enough to hold it erect without our help.

17

A word about the hands holding the child.

It is through our hands that we speak to the child, that we communicate.

Touch is the first language.

Understanding comes long after feeling.

Among blind people, touching has all its subtlety and importance.

Immediately, we sense the importance of such contact, and the importance of the way we hold a child.

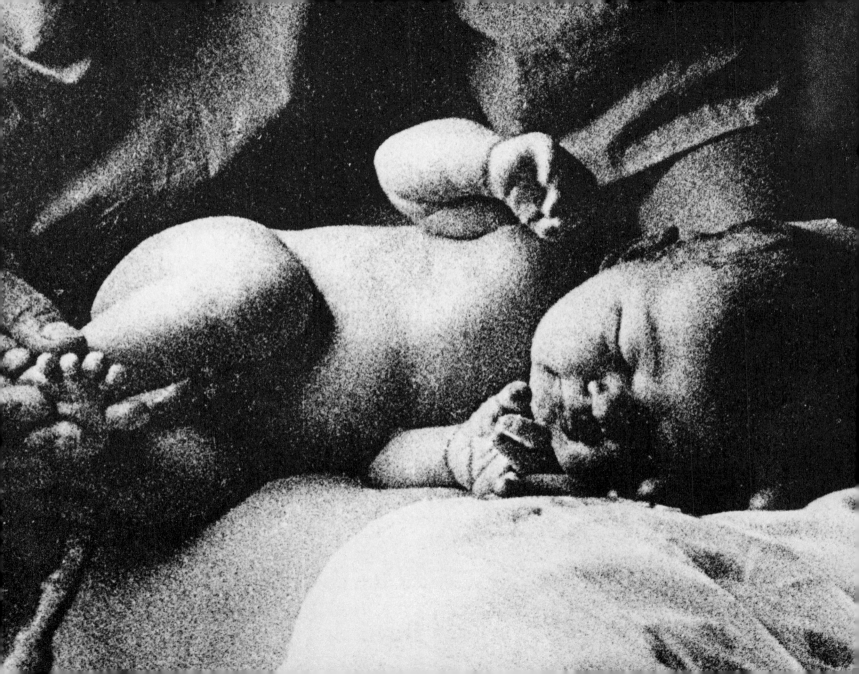

It is skin speaking to skin; and from this skin all the other sense organs derive. And these in turn are like windows in the wall of skin that contains us and holds us separate from the world.

The newborn baby's skin has an intelligence, a sensitivity that we cannot conceive of.

It is through this skin that the unborn child once knew its world, that is, its mother. It was through the whole surface of its back that it was in contact with her uterus: our backs are, literally, our past.

Now the baby is born. And suddenly this contact is gone for ever.

The baby is utterly exposed. As naked as Adam. Hands touch him. Hands, too, unlike the uterus in temperature, in weight, in the way they move, in their power, and in their rhythm.

This is the baby's first contact with the unknown, with the new world, with that which is 'other'.

And our hands that touch and hold the baby, these unknowing, unfeeling hands, have no understanding at all of what the baby has experienced until this moment.

Our hands are instruments of our intelligence, our will.

They obey muscles that are highly conscious and fast-moving. The hands' movements are sharp, sudden, almost brusque.

And terrifying to the baby who has only experienced the slow, internal rhythms of the womb.

How could the child *not* panic at this new kind of touch? So how, then, ought we to touch — to handle — a newborn baby?

Very simply: by remembering what it has just left behind. By never forgetting that everything new and unknown may terrify and that everything recognizable and familiar is reassurance.

To calm the baby in this strange, incomprehensible world into which it just emerged, it is necessary — and sufficient — for the hands holding him to speak in the language of the womb.

What does this mean?

That the hands must remember the slowness, the continuous movement of the uterine contraction, the 'peristaltic wave' the child grew to know so well during the final months before its birth.

This is another reason why it is necessary to first place the child on its stomach — so that, by massaging it, we may 'speak' to its back.

And what should our hands say? Exactly what the mother and her womb have been saying.

Not the womb as it was during the final labour, not the violent womb that expels and banishes. But the womb of the early, happy days.

The womb that pressed slowly, tenderly. The womb that embraced. The womb that was a source of love.

It was an infinitely sensual, amorous relationship that existed between the child and its mother, between the uterus and its prisoner.

What is needed is neither a brisk rubbing motion nor a caress, but a deep slow massage.

Our hands travel over the baby's back, one after the other, following each other like waves. One hand still in contact as the other begins. Each maintaining its steady rhythm until its entire journey is concluded.

Without rediscovering this visceral slowness that lovers find instinctively, it is impossible to communicate with the child.

But . . . people will say . . . you're making love to the child!

Yes, almost.

To make love is to return to Paradise, it is to plunge again into the world before birth, before the great separation. It is to rediscover the primordial slowness, the blind, all-powerful rhythm of the internal world, of the great ocean. Making love is the great regression.

What we are doing here is softening the pain of virtual exile by carrying the past forward into the present. We are giving the child company on its journey. We are soothing it by sending the echo of the familiar uterine waves along its back.

Making love is the sovereign remedy for anguish: to make love is to rediscover peace and harmony. In the cataclysm of birth is it not right that we should call upon this sovereign comfort?

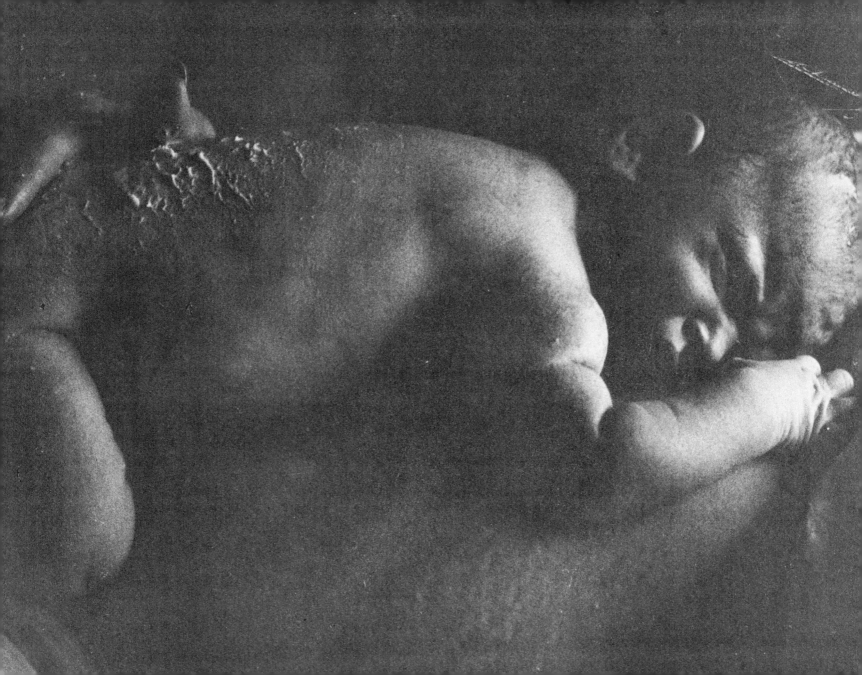

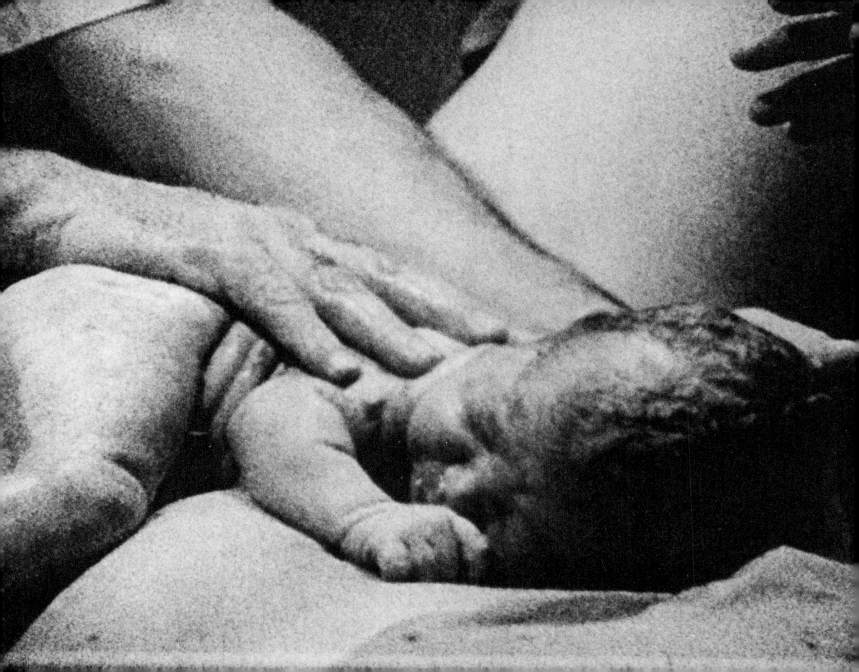

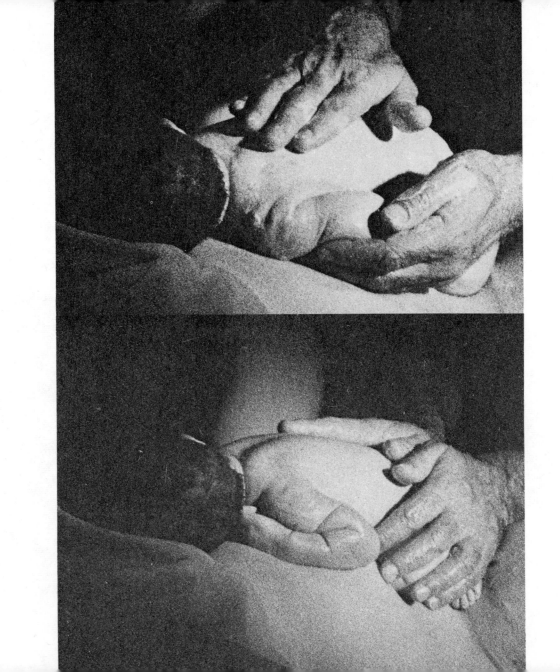

18

But our hands may also remain motionless.

The hands that touch the child reveal everything to it: nervousness or calm, clumsiness or confidence, tenderness or violence.

The child knows if the hands are loving. Or if they are careless. Or worse, if they are rejecting.

In attentive and loving hands, a child abandons itself, opens out.

In rigid and hostile hands, a child retreats into itself, blocks out the world.

So that before we even think of re-creating the pre-natal rhythms which once flowed around this small body, we must let our hands lie on it motionless.

Not hands that are inert, perfunctory, distracted.

But hands that are attentive, alive, alert, responsive to its slightest quiver.

Hands that are light. That neither command nor demand.

That are simply there.

Light . . . and heavy in the weight of tenderness. And of silence.

19

Whose hands should hold the child? The mother's, of course, provided that these hands know everything we have been saying.

This cannot be taught, although it can be forgotten.

Many mothers briskly pat their babies! Or shake them, thinking that

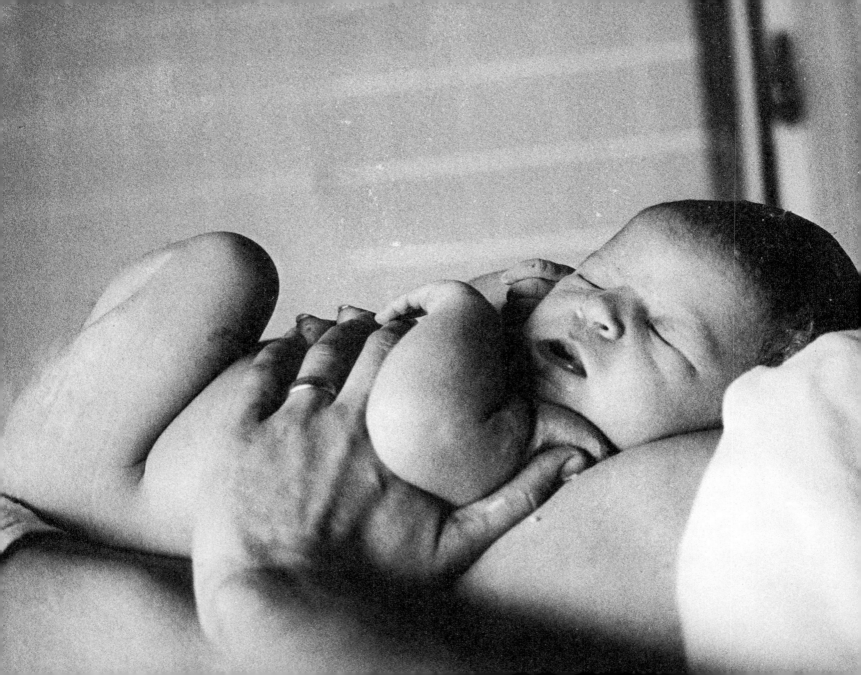

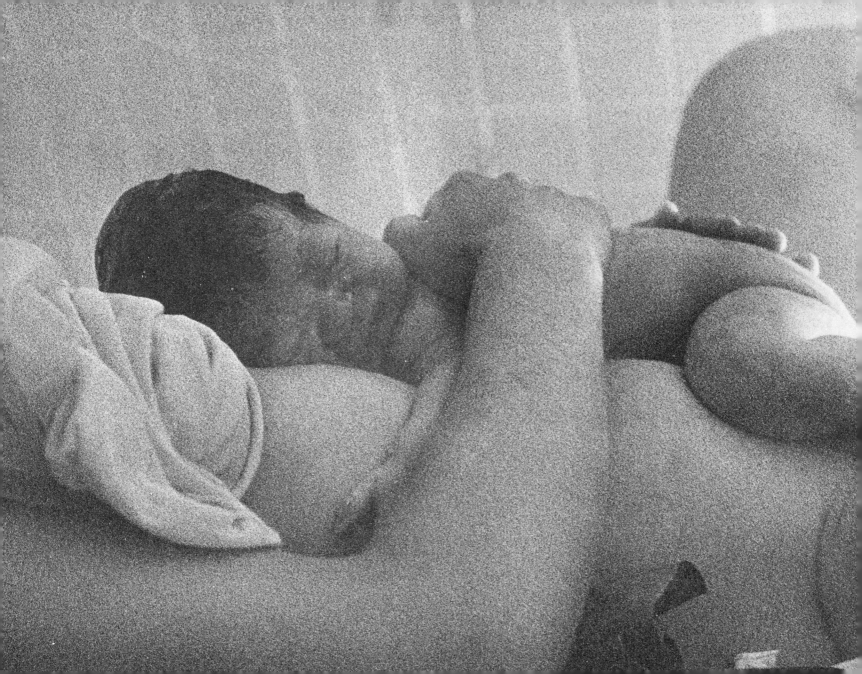

they're rocking and consoling them . . .

Many have still, lifeless, uncomprehending hands.

Many are so wrapped up in their own emotions that they are literally in danger of smothering their children.

However, in most cases the woman who has delivered her baby naturally will have had to rediscover her own body and to control its ill-timed impulses. So she is ready to hold and touch her baby.

Despite her excitement, she will not overwhelm her child.

When the newborn child is placed on her stomach, when she lays her hands on it, she will think: 'My problems are over. But not my baby's.'

The delivery is over, but the baby's awakening has just begun.

It is on the first step of a wild adventure; it is transfixed with fear.

Do not move. Do not add to the baby's panic.

Just be there. Without moving. Without getting impatient. Without expecting anything.

At this point, out of consideration for her child, out of real — not egocentric — love, a woman will simply place her hands on its body. And leave them there, unmoving. They must give a message not of excitement, agitation and emotion, but of calm and lightness, and of peace.

The wave of love that will assuage her baby's remorse can come from such hands.

20

Remorse.

Yes, remorse. Yet one more thing to surprise us.

It is easy to accept that a child can feel fear and grief. But remorse?
Nonetheless, it is so.

The idea people generally have of birth is that the child takes no personal part in it. That the child is passive, merely submitting to expulsion.

That it is the mother who does all the work.

But the reality is totally different.

The Greeks, as we know from Hippocrates, believed that it was the child who demanded to be born.

They believed that when pregnancy reached its term, the child was beginning to be short of food. Feeling its life threatened, it was forced to abandon the dark cavern which had been its home until then, and to search for the way out — using its feet to propel itself forward, to force its way towards freedom.

We have laughed at these old wives' tales, only to discover that all this is perfectly true!

We have discovered today that the stimulus that sets labour in motion comes from the child, just as the Ancients said it did. And now we know that the child actually does struggle to be born.

The speeding up of its heartbeat indicates both the enormous effort it is making and the terror it feels. And an alert mother, conscious of what is happening within her body, recognizes the exact moment when her child, doing its part, begins its desperate exertions.

So the child struggles fiercely, for its life. And it is a fight to the death. One party, mother or child, must lose.

And when the child does emerge — when the battle is won — its mother is suddenly gone.

The child feels intolerable anguish: 'I am alive, but I have killed my mother. I am here, but my mother is gone!'

This seems incredible to us. And yet it is so. Those who have relived their birth can testify to it.

So it's vital to reassure, to pacify the child immediately.

Through her hands, unmoving but tender, the mother is saying to her baby: 'Don't be afraid. I'm here. We're both safe, you and I, we're both alive.'

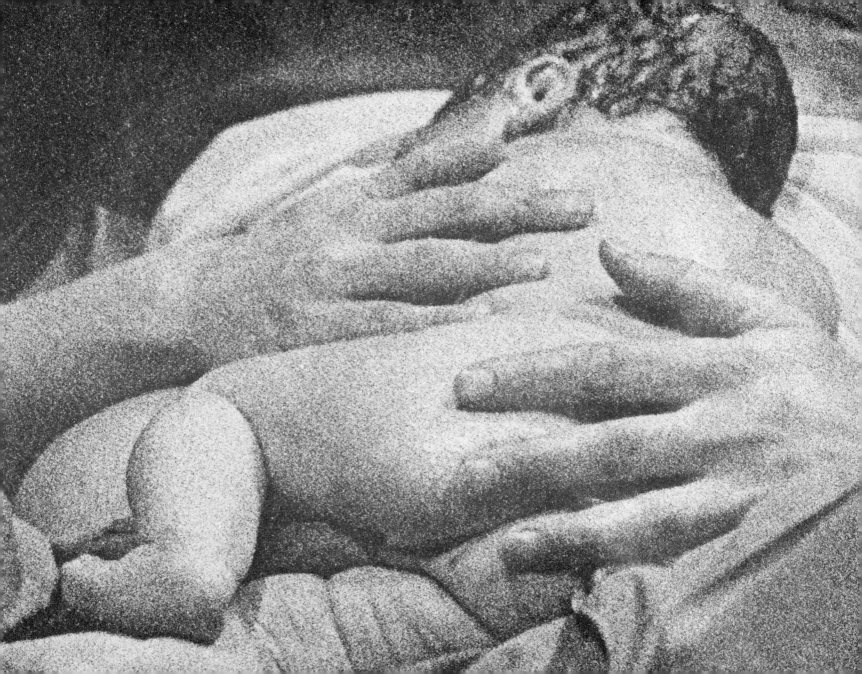

21

This first meeting between mother and child is crucial.

Many mothers do not know how to touch their babies. Or, to be more exact, do not dare. They are paralysed.

Many will not admit it, or are not even aware of it. But it is true nevertheless, if you can recognize the signs. Something restrains these mothers, some profound inhibition.

This new body has emerged from what modesty has led us to call, euphemistically, the 'private parts'.

Whatever circumlocution we use, our education has still conditioned most of us to consider these parts of the body as somehow offensive, to reject them; not to mention them.

That's where the baby has come from.

From this region of the body that we are supposed to know nothing about, that we don't examine, that we don't display or touch. That we would deny.

Now this something has emerged from 'there'. Something warm and sticky. And the result of muscular efforts that resemble those we use in excreting.

And it is this 'something' that we must touch!

Moreover, how can we place our hands on something which has just emerged from inside a human stomach? On human entrails.

The mother remains paralysed, frozen by an age-old prohibition.

Suddenly deeply confused, she no longer knows *what* she feels for this 'thing' that is there, on her belly. An immense disgust? A passionate concern?

Sometimes one has to take her hands and place them on the child.

Her resistance is obvious. But once it is overcome, once the step has been taken, the result is extraordinary.

She has transcended the taboo.

The barrier that separated her from her child, and from herself, is down.

She is filled with an indescribable joy.

The old distinction between good and bad, clean and dirty, permissible and forbidden has dissolved.

Suddenly, things are so simple. For the first time in a lifetime!

Fear has ebbed.

By touching her child, the woman has at last discovered herself. She has made herself whole.

For her, the internal and the external have been fused.

22

And now let us look again at the child, who by this time is breathing normally.

The umbilicus has been severed, all that is now far in the past . . .

Just how far? It could be years. But, measured by a watch, it is perhaps three minutes; six at the most. And yet our concentration has been so intense that we have been existing outside time.

And where exactly are we? This calm, this silence, contrast so dramatically with the shrieks that accompany so many births . . .

Just as the mothers' tranquillity during natural childbirth still has the power to amaze us, almost to unnerve, so the peace and serenity of this birth astounds us.

Yet wonderful as this calm and silence are, a still greater wonder awaits us.

The child is about to leave the mother once more.

The two have met, have rediscovered one another. Now they are going to separate.

A new step for the child on the road to freedom.

But we must take great care over this new separation. Where do we place the child? What must we do to ensure that this separation is not a shock, but a joy?

How, once and for all, do we dispel the fear that is still so close to the surface? How do we loosen all the knots of tension that may escape our eye but are revealed to the touch when we place our hands on the baby's back?

It is easy. The child is leaving the warmth and softness of its mother's stomach. We can ensure that if it finds a similar warmth and softness elsewhere.

We should not put a newborn baby on metal scales, so cold and hard.

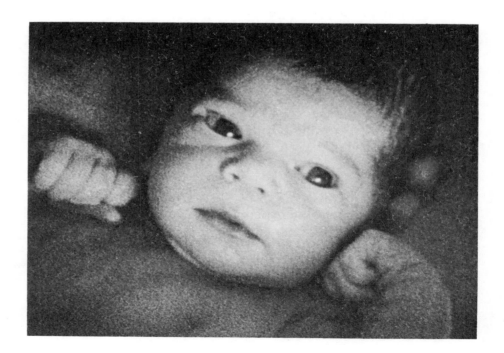

Nor in material that feels rough after the mother's smoothness and warmth.

We should place it — in fact, replace it — in water!

For the baby has emerged from water, the maternal waters that have carried it, and cradled it for so long. Made it light as a bird . . .

There should be a basin of water at hand, roughly at body temperature — ninety-eight or ninety-nine degrees.

We place the child in it.

Once again, extremely slowly.

As the baby sinks down, it becomes weightless, and is freed from this new heavy body with all its burden of harsh new sensation.

The baby floats, disembodied, light. As free as in the early, distant days of pregnancy when it could play and move about without restrictions in a limitless sea.

Its surprise and its pleasure know no bounds.

In its element once more, the baby forgets what it has just left behind; forgets its mother. Once again it is inside her.

This first separation, far from being an agony, becomes a joy.

The hands supporting the child in the bath soon feel the little body relax completely. Whatever fear, stiffness, tension might have remained now melt like snow in the sun. Everything in the baby's body that was still anxious, frozen, rigid, begins to live, to dance.

And — most wonderful of all — the child opens its eyes wide.

This first look is unforgettable.

Immense, deep, grave, intense, these eyes enquire: 'Where am I? What has happened to me?'

We feel in this baby such utter concentration, such astonishment, such depth of curiosity, that we are overcome.

We discover that, beyond any doubt, a *person* is there, someone who had been hidden behind fear and whose eyes had been held shut by terror.

We see (and it should have been obvious) that far from being a beginning, birth is just transition. And that this creature who is looking

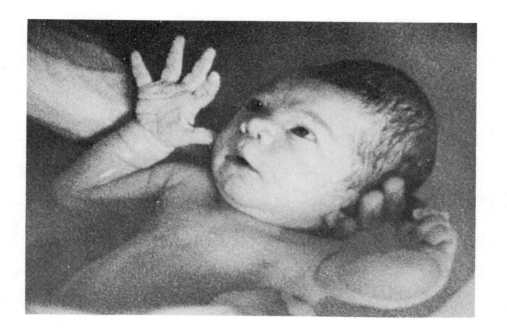

at us and questioning us has already been in existence for a long time.

Everyone who has been present at these births, who has seen these babies open their eyes, who has felt the weight of their curiosity — everyone has said with the same disbelief: 'But . . . it's not possible . . . that baby can see!'

Babies do not 'see' in our sense of the word; they don't receive images as we receive them.

But that they communicate in their own way, in a way that we have almost totally forgotten, is something which no longer can be doubted.

'A newborn baby is blind, it doesn't hear anything, feel anything. It's not yet conscious. How could you think that at that age...?'

Before the questioning intensity of these eyes, such an attitude may make us smile. And fill us with shame.

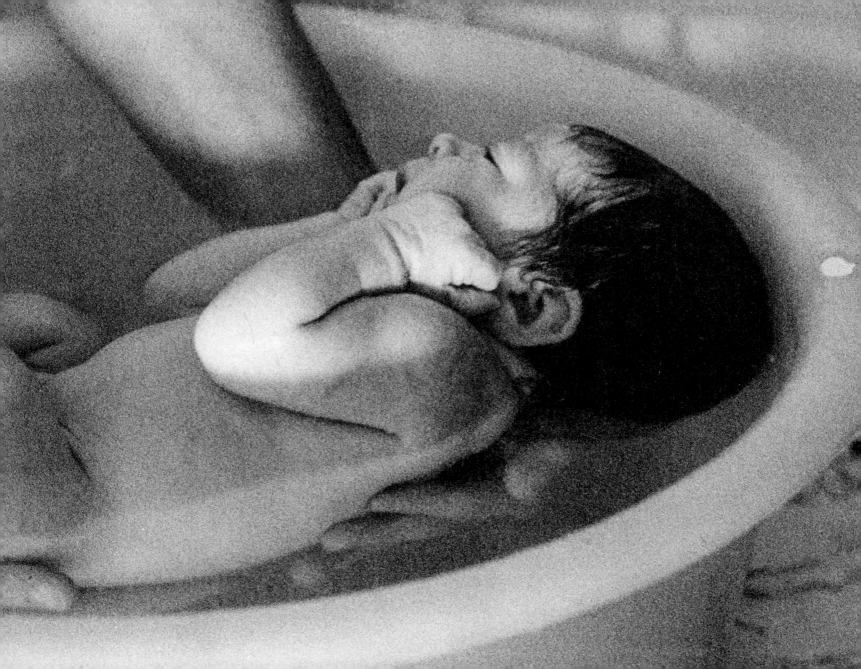

23

And what happens next is no less amazing.

Having moved from immediate fear and shock at its new condition to an acceptance of it, the child starts to explore its new domain.

Everything begins to move.

The head turns slowly to the right, then to the left, twisting around as far as the neck will allow.

A hand stirs — opens, closes — and emerges from the water.

The arm follows, rising. The hand strokes the air, feels the space around it, falls back into the water.

The other hand rises in its turn, traces a curve, retires.

Now they play together, meet, grasp and separate.

One moves away, the other darts after it.

One pauses, dreams, opens and closes with an underwater slowness. The other falls under the same spell. The two dreams mirror each other; the hands are like flowers about to blossom. Sea-anemones, they breathe with the slow cradling rhythm of the world beneath the ocean, drifting in its invisible currents.

The legs — timid at first, and unwilling to enter the game — begin moving too. Abruptly, a foot shoots out. And then the other, hitting the edge of the tub, propelling the whole baby backwards. It is beginning to enjoy itself.

It does it again.

The child is playing!

Less than ten minutes after birth.

This entire performance is taking place in total silence, punctuated only by soft little cries — exclamations of surprise and joy.

Sometimes solemn, sometimes playful, completely absorbed in its

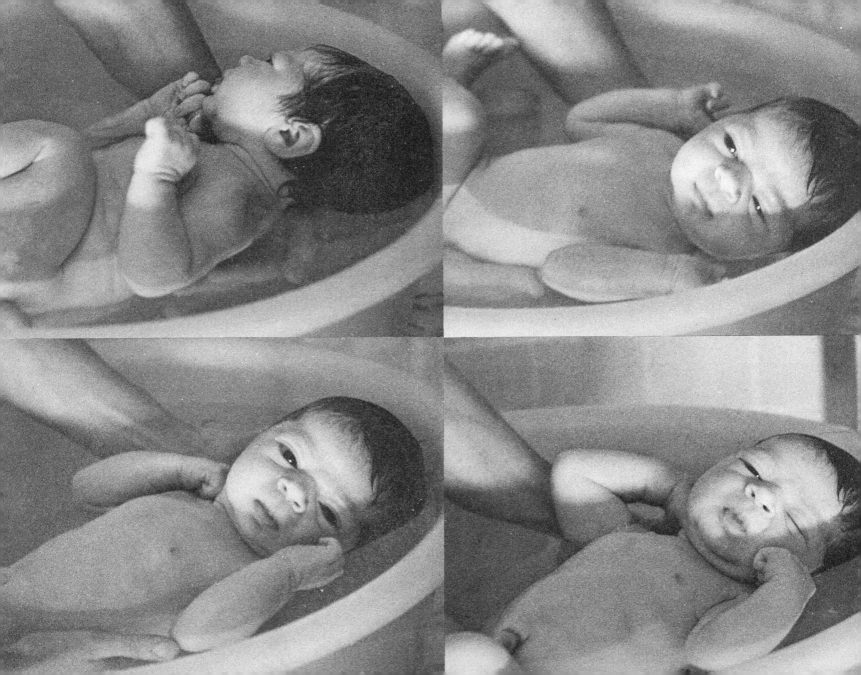

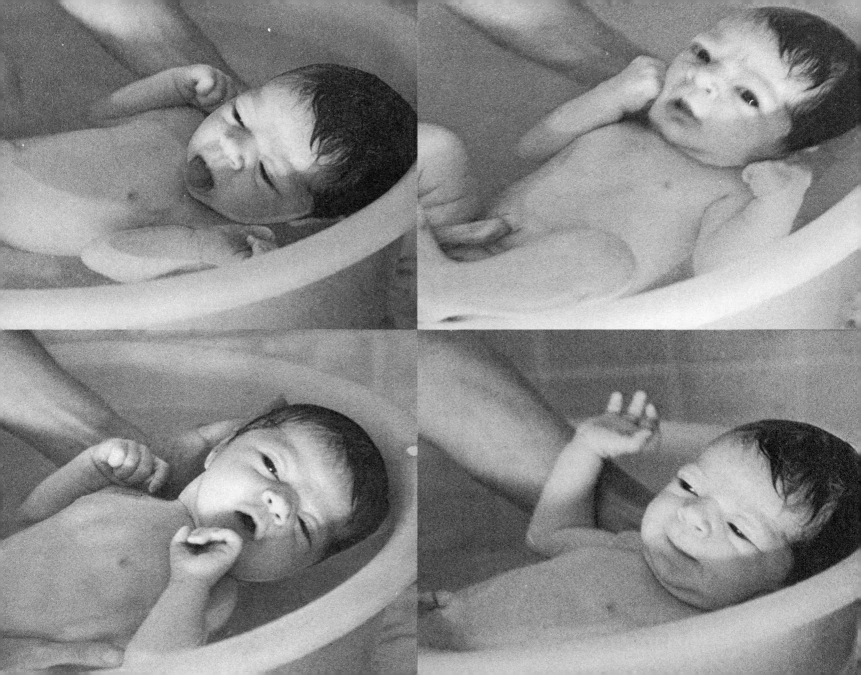

discoveries, the child explores, tests the space above, below, around it, with a concentration that never falters, that never succumbs to distraction.

Totally *there,* an impassioned observer of its own body.

It is clearly a happy child: it is a unity, a continuity, a totality. Not an inch of its body is alien to its movements. Every inch of this child is moving, living together in the most complete harmony.

How can we fail to envy this baby, we who are so fragmented, who have lost this primal unity? We who always are — or would be — elsewhere? We who are incapable simply of 'being there'?

And now the face begins to come alive. The mouth opens, closes. The lips part. The tongue pokes out and disappears. And when finally, as if by accident, a hand encounters the face, slides over it and finds the mouth, the child pushes a thumb into it and sucks delightedly.

The hand moves on. Travels once more through space, and returns to this paradise, the mouth.

This time the child would like to get its whole hand inside . . .

How could the child possibly regret the past?

Doubtless there are enemies lurking; hunger, for instance, which has not yet made its dire appearance.

It doesn't matter. Everything has begun so well that the child will enjoy a taste for adventure — for ever.

How long should we leave the child in its bath? It is for the child to decide.

We should be sure the relaxation is complete, that there isn't the least resistance in the small body, the least hesitation or tension, the slightest stiffness, the merest knot, the shadow of a doubt.

We must be sure that everything is flowing; that everything is joy.

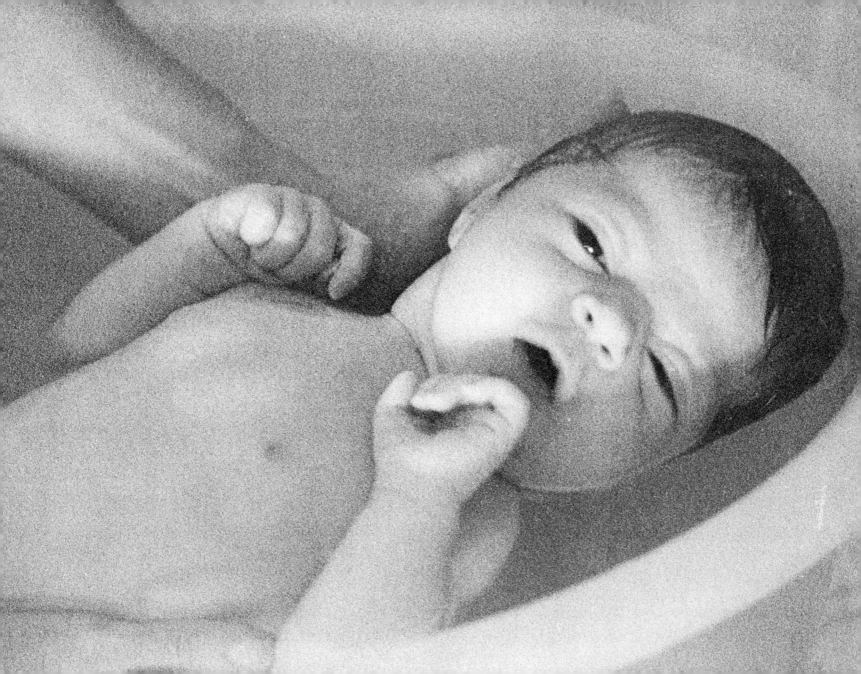

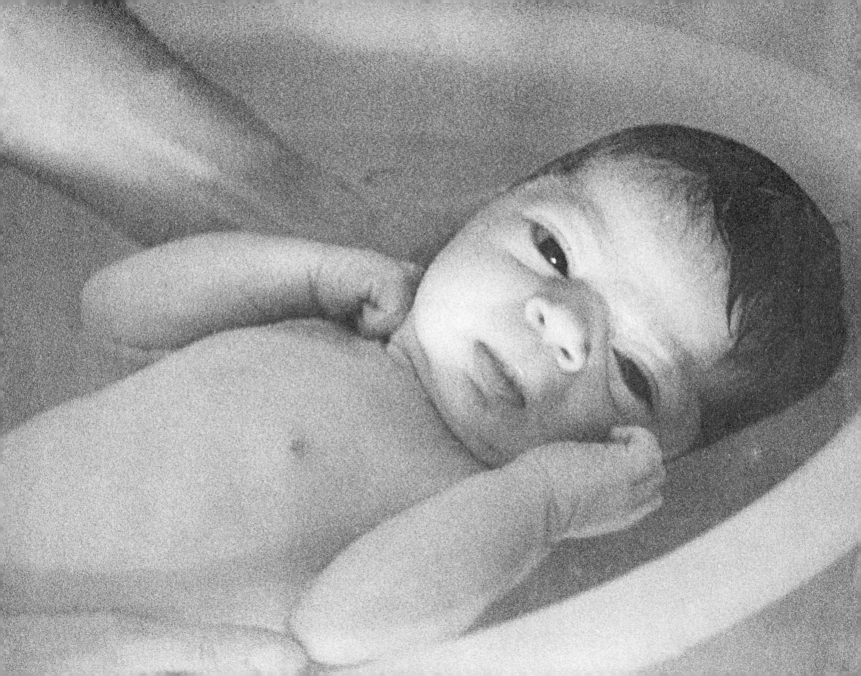

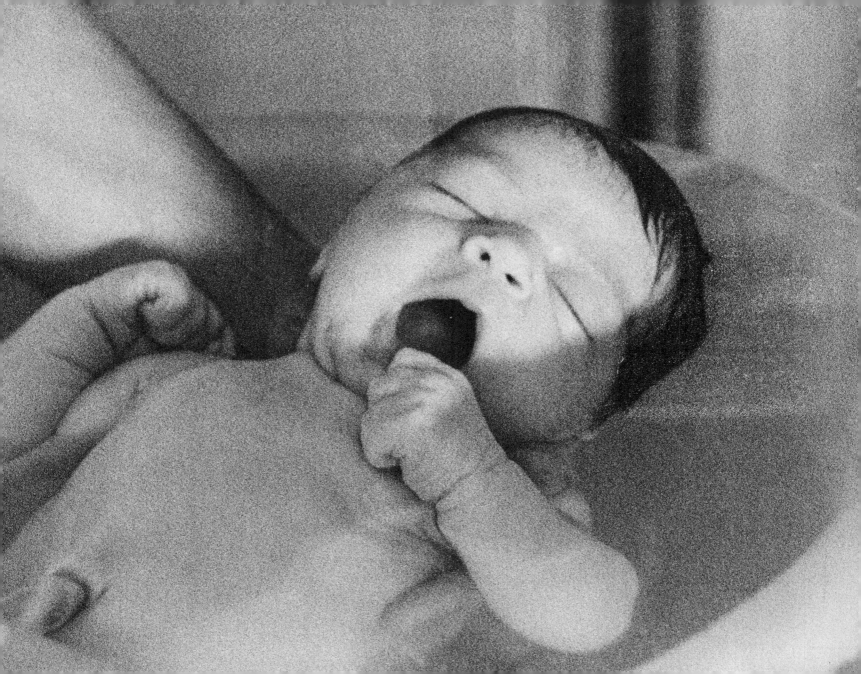

24

Now that all fear has been dispelled, now that birth and all that came before it are forgotten, it is time to emerge at last from the comforting water.

Time for the baby to take its place on terra firma.

The fourth step in the path of birth. The fourth stage.

The baby is going to be born yet again into its new element. But this time, of its own accord.

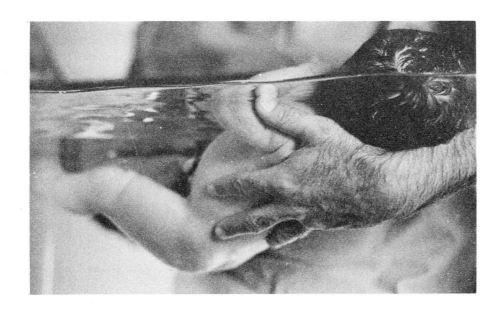

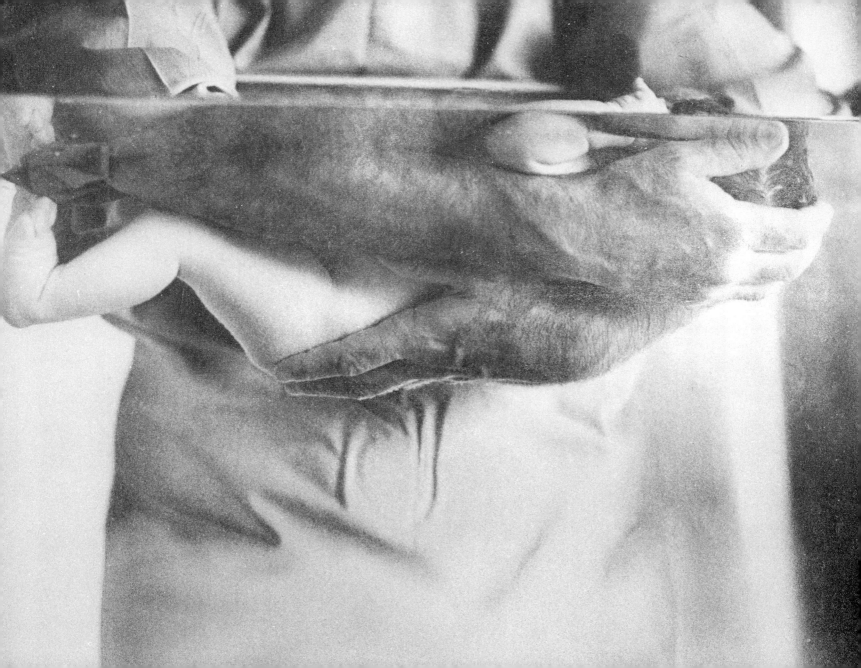

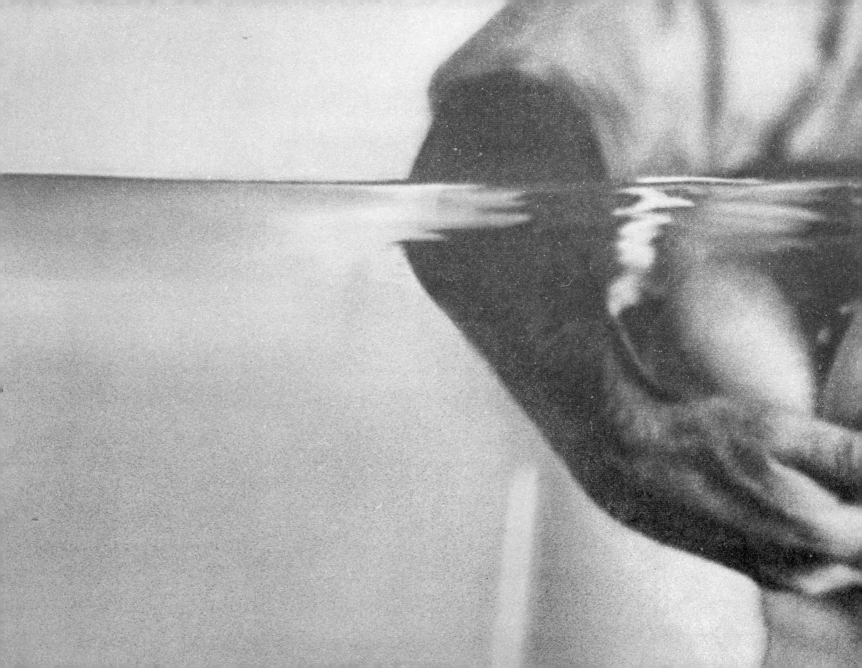

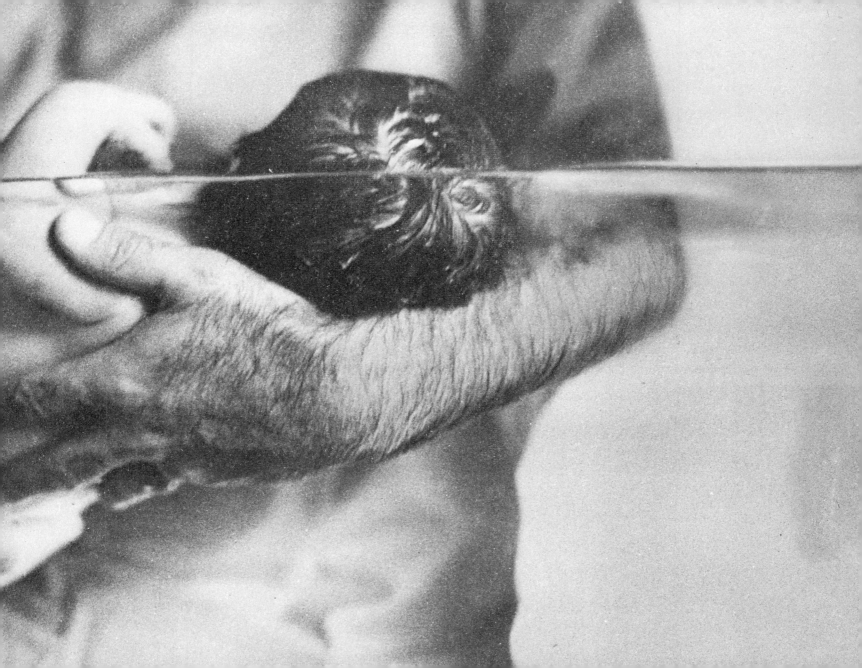

Leaving the water, the baby finds its new master, a tyrant: the weight of gravity; the new burden of its own body.

If a baby is not to be overcome by this, if it is to accept these new bonds readily, things must once again become a game. The baby must enjoy itself. So we lift it slowly from the water — as slowly as formerly we immersed it. It re-discovers its body's weight — and cries out. We put it back in. Its body is gone again! We take it out once more.

A powerful sensation, and one that is now no longer new, it has become as pleasurable as it is now familiar. So powerful and so pleasurable that every child ever born longs to experience it again.

At home with itself now, enjoying the world it is to live in, the baby is now ready to end its bath.

Now we can lie it on a napkin, ready-warmed.

We wrap it in layers of cotton and wool — the world is a cold place. We cover neither the head nor the hands, which must be free to move and play.

We place the baby on its side, *not,* of course, on its back.

Its arms and legs can move easily; its abdomen can expand and contract as it breathes; its head can turn freely.

We have taken care to put something round the baby's back, so that it senses something there, and is reassured.

And then we leave the baby to itself.

The fifth step, the fifth stage in the path of birth. For the first time the child is alone. It now discovers immobility. An extraordinary experience.

And terrifying, once again, in its utter strangeness.

For nine months, the baby has been an eternal traveller. Its shifting world has never ceased to move. Sometimes gently, sometimes violently. Its mother's body was always in motion; and even when she was still or asleep, there was always the great rhythm of her breathing, of her diaphragm.

The baby has lived in perpetual motion.

Now, a truly appalling change; everything stops.

For the first time.

Nothing moves.

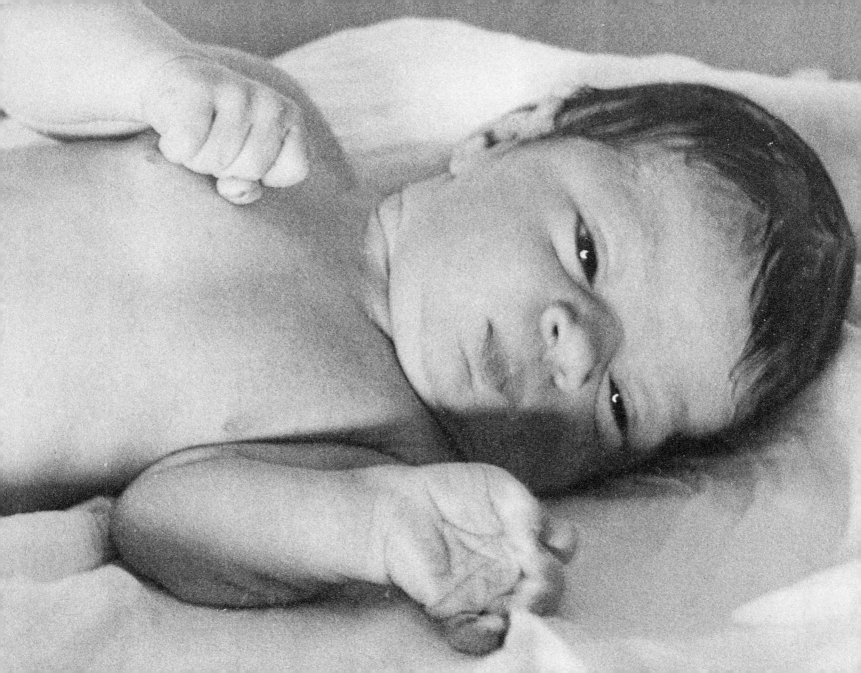

The world has frozen, died.

This is unknown territory.

A baby brought into the world the conventional way is seized by panic at this point, begins to howl in its terror and bewilderment.

Later on, every time it is reminded of this sudden sense of total immobility, of this solitude, the same panic will seize it again, and it will start to scream again, its anguish stemming not so much from being left alone as from believing that the world is once again dead. Frozen into immobility.

Then someone will cradle the baby, and it will re-encounter the beloved but accursed storm of motion, and will be appeased. It will relive the first moment of its life, preceeding from agony to agony, every time that it is picked up, held, put down again and left alone.

But our baby is free from fear. It will have gone from change to change, from one discovery to the next, so slowly, so lapped in love and care, that everything that happens is accepted with confidence and happiness. Nothing can alarm it now.

At the very moment when other newborn babies are beginning to scream and sob more violently than ever, our baby remains silent.

At this moment of transformation, our baby can close its eyes and utter a single cry.

A cry of surprise.

But not those desperate, heart-rending sobs. Never panic, never fear.

At most, a cry of anger — the baby objecting to the end of its pleasure.

Protesting against the bath being over. Expressing itself.

But discovering another, greater pleasure; experiencing something still more extraordinary. Our baby re-opens its eyes. Grows quiet. And — in silent astonishment — tastes the unknown: stillness.

The world of perpetual motion has become the world of constant stability. The storm has permanently abated; the child has reached the sea of tranquillity.

At present, it is utterly lost in the joy of discovery. Movement has not

84

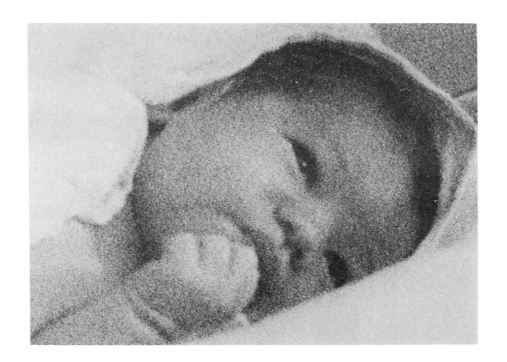

ceased; it is no longer outside, but within.

The child is moving all the time.

The eyes remain wide open, absorbed. The arms and legs continue their dance. The hands endlessly explore.

The mask of fear has disappeared for ever.

Now we are on firm ground. Our odyssey has ended.

The other monsters which await us may materialize — hunger; all the thousand natural shocks that flesh is heir to. We shall know how to counter them.

The quiet, newborn baby radiates the most intense peace.

Completely awake, supremely alert, this baby glows.

It is the child-king, the holy child referred to in the scriptures: 'Except ye be as little children . . .'

And try Lao Tse: 'The one whose grace abounding overflows, the perfect one, resembling the newborn child.'

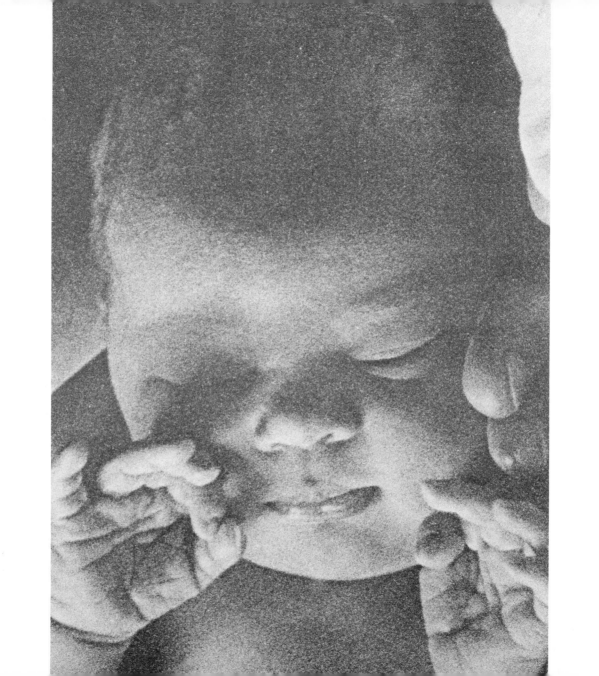

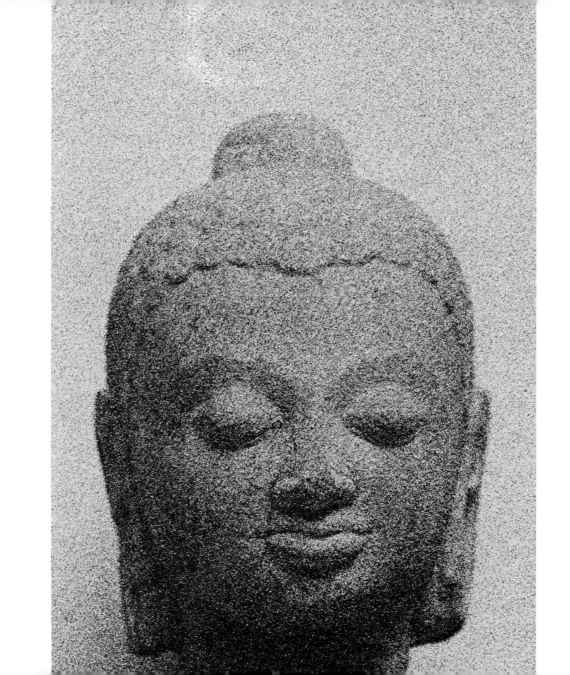

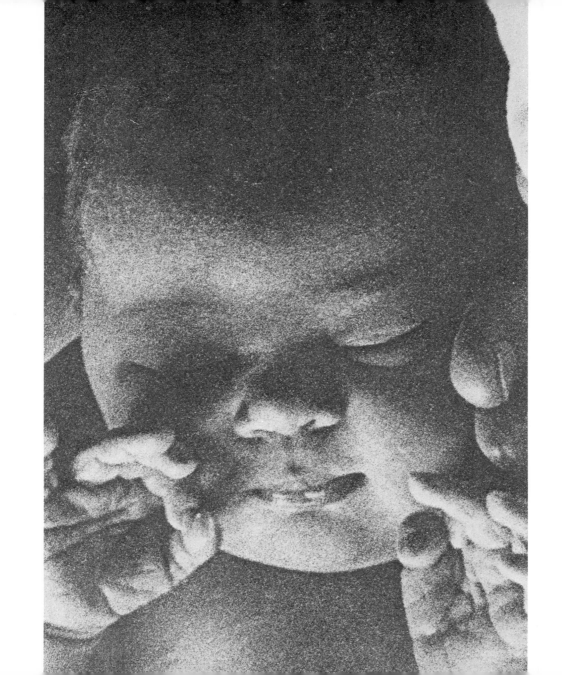

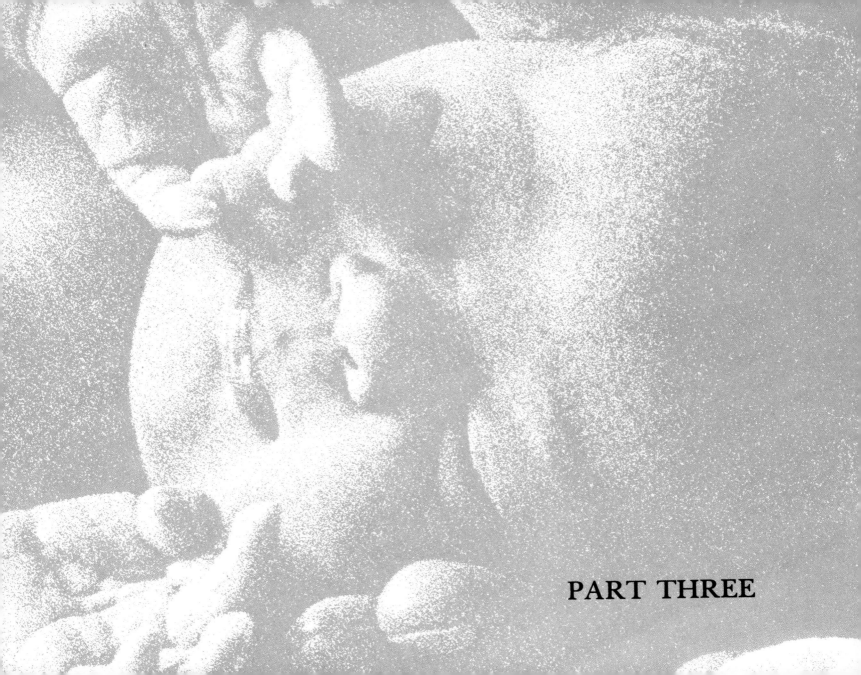

PART THREE

In the pursuit of learning, everyday something is acquired
In the pursuit of Tao, everyday something is dropped.

Less and less is done
Until non-action is achieved.
When nothing is done, nothing is left undone.

The world is ruled by letting things take their course.
It cannot be ruled by interfering.

Tao Te Ching

1

And now we shall leave this baby and return for a while to its mother, now that it has tasted the joys of solitude and stillness.

Lying once more on its mother's body, its ear against her heart, the baby re-discovers the familiar steady beat.

All is accomplished. All is perfect.

These two who have battled so fiercely are at one with each other again.

And we too are satisfied: we have understood.

We wanted to know why it was that birth was so appalling.

We said: 'If only we could understand what these newborn babies are telling us so angrily . . . What they are telling us with their flailing arms and legs, with their heads, their hands, their backs — with their screams.'

They are telling us: 'I am in pain, I am suffering.'

And even more desperately: 'I am frightened.'

The fear and the pain are one.

They are trying to express exactly what their mothers were saying, too — though without daring to be too blunt.

Who is natural and unself-conscious enough to dare to say: 'I am afraid'?

Women *didn't* dare.

But their bodies proclaimed it! The bodies of women in labour were a mass of spasms, tensions, frantic heavings, locked muscles. Their bodies sought only to escape, to deny what was taking place; they bore silent witness to their panic and terror.

Exorcizing this fear has freed women from the agony of childbirth, so that now, at times, it can become almost an ecstasy.

By sparing the child this terror, we can transform birth into enchantment.

2

To protect newborn children from fear, we must reveal the world to them infinitely slowly, and not overwhelm them with more new sensations than they can absorb and cope with.

In doing this, it is essential to reinforce memories and impressions of the past; to forge a link between past and present; to ensure that in this totally unknown, antagonistic universe, some familiar thing is there to reassure and console.

Let us try to imagine again what it is that makes this rite of passage so appalling.

Our adult senses have lost that first acuteness, that first total sensitivity. But, more important, they have become compartmentalized, and each works on its own.

Sophisticated systems filter and organize our sense impressions into coherent perceptions, give them logic and meaning. And this conditioning is so ingrained in us that we are no longer conscious of it.

Our conditioning, our *language,* hide variety from us, and protect us from the overpowering multiplicity of things.

But this is not so with the newborn baby.

Sensation is total, neither filtered nor organized.

An awkward movement, a moment of inattention, of over-eagerness, and all is lost.

The child begins to cry.

3

We have also asked: 'What is it that keeps us from seeing this new being in its separate reality?'

We know now that the answer is ourselves. It is 'I', the ego, our conditioning. What we are.

Our custom of cutting the umbilicus only moments after the baby has been born is a remarkable instance of our blindness.

'How is it', we ask ourselves, 'that Man, a rational animal of reputed intelligence, acts so irrationally at so important a moment?'

Why do we do it?

Anyone present at a birth is bound to be deeply disturbed — whether obstetrician or midwife, whether having witnessed ten births or ten thousand.

No doubt this is because we have all experienced birth. There are echoes of it deep inside us, as powerful as they are suppressed.

Nothing is forgotten — birth least of all. Only its immediate imprint has been blurred.

Thus the doctor and midwife find themselves profoundly but unconsciously involved in every birth in which they participate.

There is an unconscious change in our breathing in moments of great emotional tension.

As the climax of every delivery approaches, this emotion intensifies.

Do we realize how infectious this is, and how it feeds upon itself?

When the child makes its first appearance, emotion is at its height. And everyone's breathing — already tense — stops altogether.

'Will the baby breathe?'

Everyone is holding their breath. Identifying with the baby, however unconsciously.

We have all *returned* to our own births — fighting for breath just like this newborn baby; on the verge of suffocation.

We have no umbilicus to supply us with oxygen. So things soon become unbearable, and we feel we must take some action.

The easiest, the most sensible, the most obvious thing for the onlooker to do would be simply to breathe.

Instead of which, he cuts the baby's cord.

His own emotional involvement has made him quite irrational.

Naturally, the baby shrieks.

Everyone present exclaims in relief: 'It's breathing.'

But in fact, it is just they themselves who have found relief.

What they should really be saying is: '*I* am breathing!'

Because the truth is that the baby was in no hurry — its umbilicus gives it plenty of time.

Under the pretext of helping this new foreign being, the obstetrician has considered only himself.

Without knowing it, he has made a transference. He has rid himself of his own anguish by projecting it on to the child.

And so the victim, deprived of its umbilicus, finds itself choking for breath.

And shrieking . . .

So that we can breathe freely.

This process of transference will be endlessly repeated. And the sum of these repetitions is what we, in our ignorance, call education.

4

What remains unsaid?

At the risk of being tedious, we must return yet again to the baby's cry — the cry that was our point of departure.

'Must the baby cry?'

This question is of paramount importance. Too much is at stake here to risk misunderstandings.

The answer is clear and simple: 'Yes, the child must cry.'

And it is essential that the cry be what is called 'a good cry'. Resonant, vigorous. A clear cry in which the baby's whole body participates.

This cry — this total bodily response — confirms that all is well.

If the child is born stunned, if it is limp, if it is waiting instead of crying, every step should be taken *instantly* to produce a sharp, satisfactory cry.

This much is obvious — and there should be no possibility of misunderstanding.

In the same way, if the child coming into the world is being strangled by its umbilicus, we should not hesitate for an instant to cut it and set the baby free.

All this is common sense. Just as one wouldn't train a woman for natural childbirth when it was certain she required a Caesarean.

Perhaps it may seem that in these few lines we have negated everything we have said until now.

Not at all.

The child has to cry when being born.

Once. Or twice.

And that is enough.

Then the child must breathe. Or if it cries, then its cries must be those of strength, of vitality, of gratification.

Not cries of pain, of terror, of desolation.

No wails! No sobs!

You don't need to have a particularly sensitive or trained ear to tell the difference. You only need to be properly attentive to recognize the large and varied range a newborn baby's voice already possesses, and to see how many things it can tell us without speaking.

It only takes the slightest concentration to differentiate between the cry of life, the cry of satisfaction, and the cry of sorrow, of pain, the cry of fear.

This being so, can every child enter life as peaceably as the one we have described?

Is it possible that all of them need utter only a cry or two and then begin to breathe and murmur softly?

Certainly not.

Any more than one can promise every woman that natural childbirth will work for her.

In both experiences, anything can happen.

Each person is different. Each is unique, mysterious, unpredictable.

Sometimes a woman who seems to be physically unsuited will astonish us, while another, whose physique seems ideal, comes up against unexpected difficulties.

In the same way, each child arrives among us with its own temperament and character and heredity; its own destiny.

Each reacts in its own way. And it is amazing to see how uniquely different each one is.

Two newborn babies don't resemble each other any more than an Eskimo and a Papuan do.

And yet . . .

Curiously, during the first moments, all newborn babies are alike. For a brief period, it is still as if they had no identity at all.

Identity will come quickly. Soon it will no longer be possible to confuse them. But during those first few moments, they have a disturbing likeness.

It is simply that they all wear the same mask. The depersonalizing mask of terror.

And it is only when this mask falls away that we discover the individual beneath.

Although every child is unique, each must pass through the same stages leading from the enclosed world to the open one, from being folded in on itself to reaching outwards.

Each baby travels this path in its own manner.

And it is not necessarily those who travel it most quickly who will fare best.

Some babies seem to bound into life, then suddenly withdraw into their own anger.

Others go on struggling, eyes tight shut, failing to realize that their ordeal is over, that they have been born. It is immensely difficult wresting them from their nightmares, from their fears.

Others emerge quite casually, barely utter a cry, open their eyes and begin to play!

Still others make their way slowly, calmly, majestically. Generally speaking it is when the child has opened its eyes that the battle is over and won.

It is then, really, that he is born.

98

5

But is birth really so important? people may ask.

It doesn't last long, in comparison with what precedes and follows. It's just a nasty moment to be got through.

That, I think, is somewhat glib. After all, there is another 'nasty moment' which, though possibly equally brief, nonetheless casts a long shadow: that of death.

Birth may be a matter of a moment. But it is a unique one.

To be born means to begin to breathe, to embark on that perpetual motion which will be with us till we die.

Our breathing is the fragile vessel that carries us from birth to death.

Everyone breathes.

But there are many ways of breathing.

Whether breathing is free or impaired makes all the difference. Many people go through life half-strangled! Incapable of a real sigh, much less a real laugh!

To live freely is to breathe freely. Not just with the shoulders or the chest, but with the abdomen, with the sides, with the back.

To live and breathe fully requires a straight back, a free spinal column. Supple and live and flexible.

Many go through life with a broomstick for a spine.

The mentally ill, for instance, are incapable of breathing deeply. TALK ABOUT GLIB

If there is the least blockage along the spine, breathing — *life* — is impaired. And the person is crippled for ever. Breathing begins at the moment of birth, as do its potential failings.

Just as no two people have the same face, there are no two identical patterns of breathing. Every human being breathes in their own way. Badly, usually.

Many people acknowledge this when they say: 'I can't breathe properly, I should learn.'

Some people even try.

But it is not a thing that can be learned.

Your way of breathing was established — once and for all — at the moment you were born.

Later is too late. It should have been thought about *then*.

6

More dangerously, others will say: 'Doubtless birth does mark the child, but life is no game. It's a merciless battle. A jungle. So, like it or not, aggressiveness is essential.'

It is a total error to imagine that birth without violence produces children who are passive, weak, slow. Quite the contrary.

Birth without violence produces children who are strong, because they are free; without conflict. Free and fully awake.

Aggression is not strength. It is exactly the opposite. Aggression and violence are the masks of weakness, impotence and fear.

Strength is sure, sovereign, smiling.

It will be hard work convincing the advocates of aggression.

They themselves have suffered, and so they say: 'Life has been hard for me. I've been knocked around, and it's made me what I am. Let it be the same for my children.'

Really what they are saying, without admitting it, is: 'I've suffered. Why shouldn't others suffer too?'

The dreadful law of reprisal.

These are the people who used to say (or who even now still say): 'Women suffer in childbirth. All right, that must be because they have to.'

This is frightful, *a posteriori* logic. We know what people really mean by all the musts of this kind. They are really talking about evil, sin and atonement. The cult of suffering is not new. It leads directly back to the stake, to the Inquisition, to all the massacres committed in the name of king or conscience.

There is no sin involved here.

There is only error and ignorance. Our blindness and our resignation. This kind of suffering is pointless. It serves no purpose.

It satisfies no god. It springs from a failure of intelligence.

Natural childbirth — childbirth without pain — stands as proof of this.

7

After all this, I can say only one thing: 'Try.'

Everything that has been said here is simple. So simple that one feels embarrassed at having dwelt upon it at such length.

Perhaps we have lost our taste for simplicity.

Here, we need so little. None of these expensive gadgets for monitoring, none of the technologist's modish products.

Only a little patience and humility. A little silence. Unobtrusive but real attention. Awareness of the newcomer as a person. Unself-consciousness.

And love.

Without love, the delivery room can be perfect — lighted only as strongly as necessary, the walls soundproofed, the bath temperature at just the right degree — and still the child will scream.

If there's still some trace of nervousness, some ill-humour or impatience, some suppressed anger, the baby will sense it.

Its judgment is frighteningly sure.

The baby knows everything. *Feels* everything.

The baby sees right into our hearts, knows the colour of our thoughts.

All without language.

The **newborn baby** is a mirror, reflecting our image. It is up to us to see it doesn't cry.

8

'There's something you haven't mentioned.'

'What?'

'These children, born in silence and love — what becomes of them? Are they different from others?'

'It's hard to say. You have to see them.'

'Well . . .?'

'Sometimes, when the baby is born it wears a mask which hides it, disfigures it, makes it ugly . . . The mask of tragedy — brows knitted, corners of mouth turned down . . . But there is another mask. A mask of gaiety, of joy — a comic mask. With a wide mouth lifted into a smile. With eyebrows relaxed, and eyes crinkled with pleasure. . .'

'But surely *that* mask has never been seen on a newborn baby. It's impossible.'

'You think so? Look . . .'

'Oh! That baby isn't smiling — it's *laughing!* It's positively hooting!'

'You said it, not me.'

'How marvellous . . . but this hasn't anything to do with what we've been discussing.'

'And why not?'

'We've been discussing birth and newborn babies. You're showing me a child six months old.'

'Six months old?'

'Babies don't smile before two months. One and a half at the earliest. As for laughing aloud . . .'

'That's what people say. But *this* baby isn't even twenty-four hours old!'

102

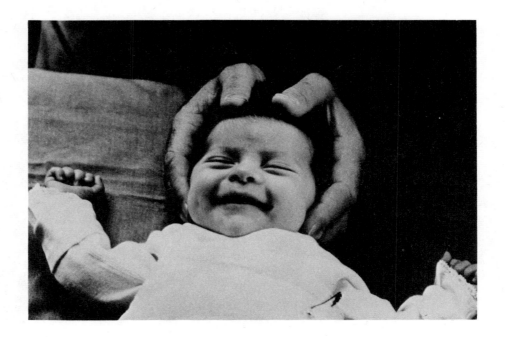

'I can't believe it!'

'I admit it doesn't happen very often, at least not yet. But . . . do you know that there's still another mask? Or rather a *real* face without any mask at all?'

'I don't understand.'

'Our emotions are states of mind — impermanent, always changing. We cherish some of them, others we fear. But in reality they are all one. Laughter and tears are very close. And this joy which astonishes you in one baby is ultimately no more remarkable than another baby's sorrow. It is still only a mask.'

'But what can be left when the child is without a mask? What is there when both joy and sorrow have disappeared.'

'Almost nothing. Look . . .'

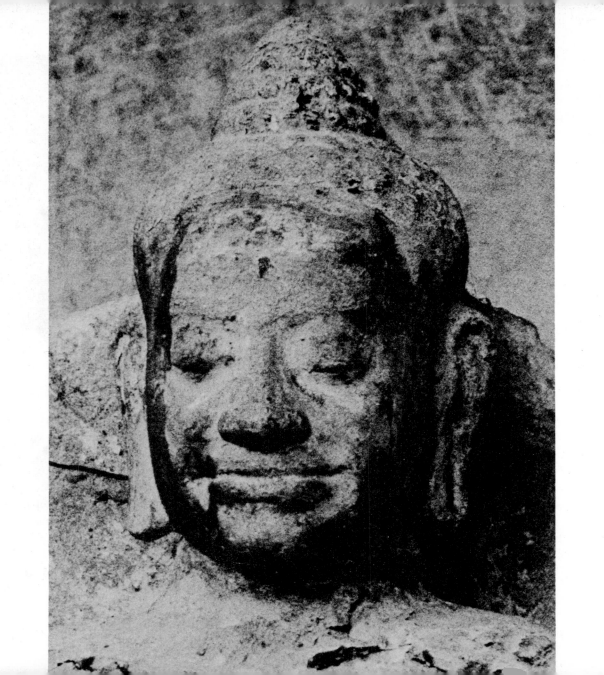

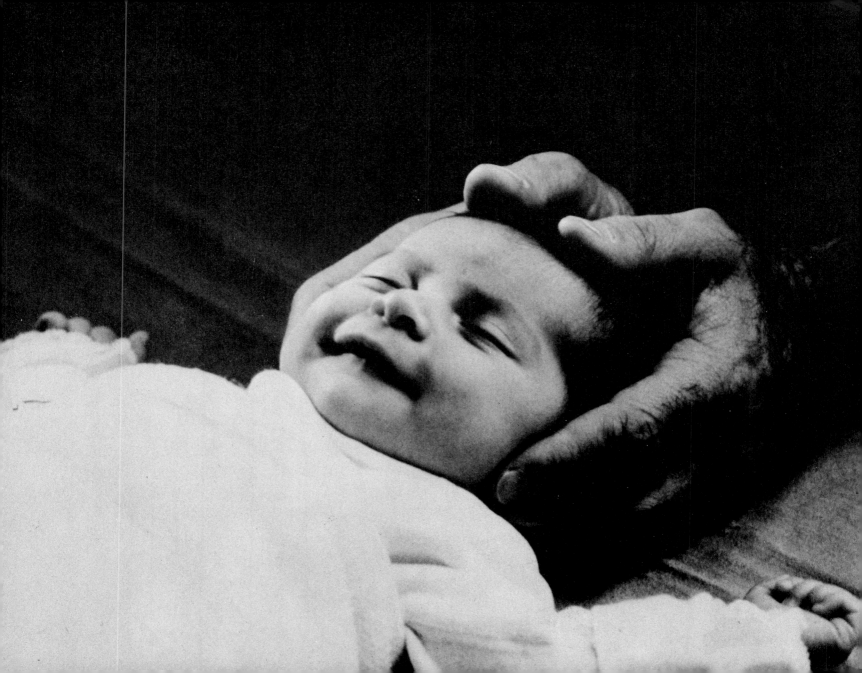